New Perspectives on Medical Clowning

Taking the recent coronavirus pandemic as a starting point, this book presents and analyzes new research around medical clowning in hospitals, from social media use to the impact on the hospitalized child in later life.

This innovative book begins with an overview of the work of medical clowns. It discusses the idea of humor as a mechanism related to the revolution in language and human consciousness, and makes a connection between humor and anxiety, exploring how this can be mobilized to support hospitalized patients. There is extensive examination of medical clowning to strengthen coping skills and promote wellbeing in the time of Covid-19, where loneliness and isolation loomed large and anxieties were high. Subsequent chapters explore the role of medical clowning in wartime and at time of natural disasters, the experiences of children some time after their experience of hospitalization and clowning, and the role of social media and medical clowns in community building.

This book is a fascinating contribution to the literature on medical clowning. It is of interest to researchers, practitioners, and lecturers in medical clowning, play in healthcare, nursing, medicine, and performance studies.

Amnon Raviv earned his PhD in medical clowning. He is a clown doctor in hospitals as part of the Dream Doctors project. Amnon Raviv is a Researcher and Lecturer at Ben Gurion University. He is a philosopher, musician, director, and actor.

T0325979

New Perspectives on Medical Clowning

Clown Doctors in Covid-19, Wartime, and the Everyday

Amnon Raviv

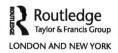
Routledge
Taylor & Francis Group

LONDON AND NEW YORK

First published 2023
by Routledge
4 Park Square, Milton Park, Abingdon, Oxon OX14 4RN

and by Routledge
605 Third Avenue, New York, NY 10158

Routledge is an imprint of the Taylor & Francis Group, an informa business

© 2023 Amnon Raviv

The right of **Amnon Raviv** to be identified as author of this work has
been asserted in accordance with sections 77 and 78 of the Copyright,
Designs and Patents Act 1988.

Trademark notice: Product or corporate names may be trademarks
or registered trademarks, and are used only for identification and
explanation without intent to infringe.

British Library Cataloguing-in-Publication Data
A catalogue record for this book is available from the British Library

ISBN: 978-1-032-42330-2 (hbk)
ISBN: 978-1-032-51544-1 (pbk)
ISBN: 978-1-003-36230-2 (ebk)

DOI: 10.4324/9781003362302

Typeset in Times New Roman
by codeMantra

Dedicated with love to my beloved children Toot and Yam and my dear parents Esther and Tuvia.

Contents

Figures

Note: All figures Courtesy of Amnon Raviv, beside 4.1, 4.2, 4.3 - Courtesy of Jan Tomasz Rogala and 4.5 Courtesy of Hagar Hofesh.

Preface – How I became a medical clown

It's all due to my mother that I became a medical clown.

Here's the story …

In my early twenties I landed in Amsterdam. I had a plan: I would buy a van, take out the back seats, put a mattress in (so I could sleep in it), and travel around Europe as a street performer. The plan succeeded: I performed with my partner during that summer and quickly discovered that the audience loved the show and was very generous. I had a lot of fun, the audience made sure that the hat was full of money at the end of the show, I met a lot of interesting people and had great experiences around the continent. There was no reason to go home at the end of the summer. The original plan of a two-month adventure turned into a four-year journey.

In those years of the mid-1980s there were no computers or mobile phones – yet, every two or three weeks I would call from the central post office of the city where I was staying (or from friends' homes) to let my parents know that I was fine, and to hear how they were doing. One day, after four years of performing, my father picked up the phone and told me in a worried voice that my mother had cancer, was operated on and was hospitalized at the Hadassah Medical Center, Ein Karem, in Jerusalem. I felt as if an arrow pierced my heart, and I boarded a flight to Israel the next day. I landed at Ben Gurion International Airport in the evening and immediately took a taxi to the hospital in Jerusalem, arriving late in the evening. Visiting hours were over, so I had to argue with the guard who was not willing to let me in. Only after examining my passport and verifying that I had indeed arrived that day from abroad did he let me in. I entered the room where my mother was lying, surprised to the core. She had no idea I was returning to see her, and barely recognized the guy who looked like a vagabond with long hair and an overgrown, bushy beard. On one shoulder was the guitar I bought from gypsies in Seville, and on the other a tall red unicycle that

I soldered together in Amsterdam from bicycle parts. On my back was a pack with some clothes and juggling equipment.

A pale and weak mother watched in disbelief. This was undoubtedly one of the most touching moments experienced by mother and son. In the weeks and months that followed, I stayed close to her, accompanying mother to the treatments, and then through a rehabilitation process, until she recovered.

The cancer "visited" her one more time, twenty years later. She also recovered from the second round, after doctors had to amputate part of her foot. We would sit before, after, and during the treatments, filling in the gaps of my four years in Europe. We mostly laughed the whole time – laughing about everything, about life, cancer, memories, and even farts. Mom and I always shared a common sense of humor and now the situation summoned the humor and laughter even more. I was her private clown and she was my first patient. The year was 1987, and, in fact, it was there under these most personal circumstances that I began my journey as a medical clown.

In the long weeks and months of accompanying my mother through the difficult oncology wards suffused with sadness, I made a decision

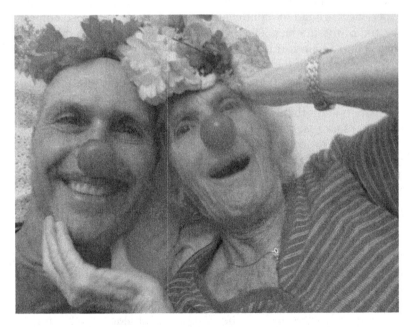

Figure 0.1 My mother and I are celebrating mother's birthday.

to enter these wards as a clown, after my mother recovered. I felt the need to enter the wards of the most seriously ill patients as a clown and musician, to bring some light and humor to patients facing the most difficult challenge of their lives.

The year before I returned to Israel to take care of my mother, a pioneering medical clown project began in New York. Clowns began visiting a children's hospital. The year was 1986, the beginning of medical clowning as a profession. I had already heard about this project from street artists who came from the USA to perform on the streets of Europe, and knew some of the clowns of the Big Apple in New York. The project sounded important to me, but the oncology wards seemed the farthest thing from the bustling streets of the European cities in which I performed. I could not guess how close they were, and could not imagine the circumstances which were about to become extremely personal (Figure 0.1).

Foreword

Dr. Amnon Raviv was the first, and so far, the only medical clown, to have earned a PhD (from the University of Haifa). His dissertation was titled *"Medical Clowning with Patients with Life Threatening and Incurable Diseases."* Raviv's first book, *Medical Clowning: The Healing Performance* (2018), combined autoethnographic descriptions of his work with children and adult patients; interviews with other clowns, patients, and hospital staff; and a discussion of medical clowning in the context of healing rituals and carnival theories. It was a tremendous contribution to what I once referred to as the "emerging profession of Healthcare Clowning."

In the current book, *New Perspectives on Medical Clowning: Clown Doctors in Covid-19, Wartime, and the Everyday,* Amnon now updates, expands, and offers insights on topics facing medical clowns: What are the challenges of achieving direct, joyous, human contact during Covid-19 or wartime? Music speaks all languages. How does it impact serious and chronic illness and what type of music has positive effects on what type of illness? How does one train to become a medical clown? How do you train to become friends with the unknown? How do smart phones and social media impact the work of medical clowns.

Quite often, people ask me: "How do you see the future of medical clowning?" My response: "We must deepen our relationship with our medical partners and in the spirit of co-creation, the future of medical clowning will unfold." We need people like Amnon very much. We need his heart, which is always available and his ability to clearly articulate the successes and challenges of our emerging profession. Emerging profession? Hmmm. Although the activity of bringing joy to various vulnerable populations will certainly continue to evolve, his current book *New Perspectives on Medical Clowning: Clown Doctors in Covid-19, Wartime, and the Everyday* is a clear indication that it has arrived. Joy finds its way.

Michael Christensen

1 Humor, consciousness, and anxiety

Many philosophers and intellectuals throughout history have tried to define, describe, and characterize humor, including Plato, Aristotle, Descartes, Hobbes, Kant, Schopenhauer, Kierkegaard, Nietzsche, Bergson, and Freud. Contemporary humor researchers tend to divide theories of humor into three main theoretical traditions based on incongruity, superiority, and release (Lippitt 1994, 1995a, 1995b, 1996).

Incongruity – Kant analyzes laughter as an incongruity of expectations, as an expectation that suddenly disappears in surprise. Incongruity can occur at the meeting between different content worlds, at the encounter between cultures with different social, conceptual, and behavioral conventions. Basically, anything that creates incongruity with our conceptual logical concepts and social conventions has a humoristic potential.

Superiority – Plato considers laughter as a flaw and an expression of ignorance, and sees laugher and mockery as negative, especially humor that results from opposition and disapproval. Nowadays, humor is seen as a positive virtue, but the humor that humiliates others (for reasons of race and skin color, for example) is negative and illegitimate. Humor and laughter have an anarchic and critical basis. Another example is satire, which mocks and criticizes political and social phenomena and has an important critical role in the sociopolitical culture of every community and society. The question is whether critical humor has been used order to oppress the individual, or whether its purpose is to vent feelings and challenge conventions to free the individual and the community from any fixed ideas and oppression. Bergson claimed that people are afraid of being mocked, and that laughter makes them perceived as ridiculed and inferior. He argues that society or government can make cynical use of the human fear of being the target of ridicule and laughter in order to impose their desires and goals on the "rebellious" individual (Lippitt 1995a).

DOI: 10.4324/9781003362302-1

Release – Freud is the main formulator of the theory. Freud claims that aggression as well as conscious and unconscious tension, breaks down in the interaction between the one who tells a joke and the one who hears the joke. The format called a "joke" allows the release of tension that naturally exists between people by converting it into shared enjoyment and interpersonal empathy. The possibility of the teller and the listener of the joke being part of each other's thought process enables an experience of shared pleasure and the release of unconscious aggression (Christoff & Dauphin 2017).

These three central theories and others shed light on certain characteristics and aspects of humor but cannot holistically present this unique phenomenon. This is similar to several people watching a huge animal with each one characterizing it from his narrow angle of vision, dictating as much as he can see. Moreover, humor changes, thus changing its meaning and function according to the increasing needs of the individual and of the community. For example, for cancer patients, humor is an internal command to fight the disease and its consequences, a weapon in the battle to live. But for the terminally ill whose fate is determined and the battle is over, humor changes its meaning and function. Instead of a weapon in the war for life, humor becomes a means by which one can arrive at acceptance, completion, and parting with the world with a smile. Humor enables embracing closure with family, friends, and the self, becoming the possibility of personal redemption.

I would like to propose a new theory of humor. I see humor as a type of alternative existential consciousness. To explain it, I need to describe how I observe the process from an evolutionary perspective.

"Language revolution" is the name commonly given by many scholars to an important evolution that took place 70,000 years ago among *Homo sapiens* (Harari 2013). Perhaps the term "revolution of consciousness" is more appropriate. Most contemporary theories see consciousness as a form of information processing (Attardo 1997). Language is probably just one of the manifestations of the revolution of consciousness, which involved the development of the brain and its ability to create a high self- and social consciousness among humans. Gervais and Sloan Wilson (Gervais & Wilson 2005) claim that humor and laughter integrated together and are intertwined in biological and social evolution. Belief, narrative, anxiety, imagination, and humor are abilities derived from a high self (and social) consciousness. As I see it, humor is an aspect of human consciousness that mediates reality in a softer and more tolerable, more entertaining way.

Human consciousness might lead to an understanding that our lives are meaningless in the perspective of eternity and cosmic space. We live on a planet that probably has no meaning in such a context and if it disappears it probably will have no consequence to the cosmos. The length of our lives and our actions as an individual and as a species seems to be negligible. This is the incongruity at the base of human consciousness. The gap between the importance of our lives in our eyes (our desire to live and leave behind something significant) and the insight of what appears to be the lack of meaning in our cosmic existence, can cause existential anxiety (among other things).

This existential anxiety must receive a mental-emotional response. One of the ways of dealing with existential anxiety is through the mechanism of humor, which enables a change of consciousness (Berk et al. 2014). Humor offers a different point of view of human existence, as well as an alternative perspective in observing reality, which allows for the reduction of anxiety and stress.

In the twilight of his life, the students of Democritus asked the Greek philosopher to summarize life from the height of his age. His response was that he could summarize life in three syllables: ha ha ha. Humor allows us to look at life in an amused way and thereby reduce our existential anxiety and the fear of death (Raviv 2018).

Another way to deal with existential anxiety is religious belief and various practices derived from the various beliefs (Malhotra & Thapa 2015). The difference between the different ways to deal with existential anxiety is that humor offers a different point of view of reality, while religious belief offers an alternative interpretation for understanding the reality. In any case, both ways offer sort of salvation from existential anxiety.

It is difficult (or impossible) to detect humor in animal behavior and certainly not in religious practice. Both humor and religion are related to the higher consciousness that is unique to humanity.

Animals think and have a simple language. Animals can communicate with different voices that warn of dangers or have a social and personal message of grief, estrus, empathy, anger, or territoriality. Voices and sounds that connect to a basic language that enables a hunter's strategy (Harari 2013). Human consciousness deals (among other things) with ontological and epistemological questions, such as the meaning of life, how we were created, the meaning of death, and the purpose of living. Man tried to understand and interpret natural phenomena. What is lightning and the sudden storm? What are the stars?

Mythologies and religions were born in order to give an interpretation and answer to the existential questions and the anxieties that accompanied them. Stories told around campfires over tens of thousands of years in the societies of hunter-gatherers were formed into mythologies passed down from generation to generation. Religions with different explanations and prayer practices shaped reality and gave meaning to people's lives and thus created order and gave answers to ontological and epistemological questions. Order, identity, and meaning provided an answer and reduced anxiety.

Along with the mythologies and religions that offered a rigid framework of identity, belonging and meaning, another cognitive mechanism was created to deal with anxiety and this mental mechanism (often referred to as sense) is humor. (A religious framework is monovalent with no room for the doubts and anxieties that arise due to the ontological and epistemological questions. The framework in itself causes anxiety).

Unlike the unquestionable rigid conceptual (and communal) frameworks offered by religions, humor offers an alternative: it is flexible, adapting itself to the character, temperament of the individual, and the need that arises in a given situation. Humor has an anarchic carnival element that challenges conventions and axioms. Unlike religion, it allows and contains different worldviews and viewpoints. Like religion, it is a tool into which one can cast positive or negative content, and, similar to religion, it can reduce anxiety and even lead to personal redemption.

Humor has several roles in our lives. Besides reducing anxiety (and sometimes even physical pain) it allows us to observe reality from an alternative and more objective point of view. It enables us to better cope; it facilitates improved, warmer interpersonal communication between people (as mentioned, not all expressions of humor are positive in their effect, as expressions of humiliating and mocking humor that have a negative effect). Humor gives us great pleasure in its various manifestations, enabling the transmission of personal, social, or political criticism in a sophisticated way.

Every time that a verbal, visual, social, existential, and conceptual situation presents an "incongruity," it has humorous potential, unless it threatens us. For example, a video from the "Candid Camera" or "stunt" genre featured a man waiting for an elevator. As soon as the elevator doors opened, he discovered a tiger tied up inside the elevator. The incongruity with his daily routine did not amuse him and he jumped back in alarm. Those who may have found the video amusing were those who watched it on their mobile or computer screen, and did not feel threatened by it (which opens a new discussion about personal taste in types of humor, as well as a discussion of ethics in humor that I will not engage in at this point).

The practice of medical clowning employs four main types of "incongruity": lowering, exaggeration, inversion, and absurdity. In most humorous situations these features of incongruity appear together in varying combinations.

Lowering – Lowering can be expressed through mockery of a character, of personal behavioral characteristics, of social or existential situations. For example, as a medical clown on the ward, I lower the characters I portray while speaking in gibberish and using accents.

Exaggeration – Exaggeration of a form of speech, saying many or few sentences in relation to what is acceptable for a given situation, or performing an excessive number or very few actions, and excessive use of objects or the objects themselves are exaggerated, excessive or reduced in their acceptable size. For example, if I wear extra-large clown shoes and dance the ballet with large and exaggerated movements.

Inversion – Inversion of what should be said or done, reversal of accepted convention, reversal of gender, hierarchy, physical, or conceptual reversal. For example – in hierarchical inversion, the clown presents himself as the head of the department; an example of gender inversion is a male clown who wears dresses.

Absurdity – The absurd is a far-fetched illogical idea that does not exist in reality, one that is not logical in action or speech, but mixes together unrelated worlds of content that have zero rational connection. For example, personifying the computer cart and dancing with it as a partner, or a clown's ride on the IV pole as if it were a scooter.

The "incongruity" of the first three types has a connection to social, cultural, and institutional conventions, and is bound by convention. This means that a certain act can be humorous and funny in a certain culture (e.g., a national or institutional culture) because it goes against conventions and creates incongruity, but the same act in another culture is unacceptable and not funny, or the opposite. For example, if in a certain society it is customary to say good morning and add an imitation of a rooster crowing, in another society this practice can be amusing because it is not acceptable.

The fourth type of incongruity is universal, and has to do with **fantasy**. Humor's link to absurdity and fantasy is of great significance in the hospital wards in the profession of medical clowning. The medical clown in the hospital wards strives to reach a connection and a strong relationship with the patient. The connection between the medical clown and the patient creates empathic humor that strengthens and empowers the patient (Figure 1.1).

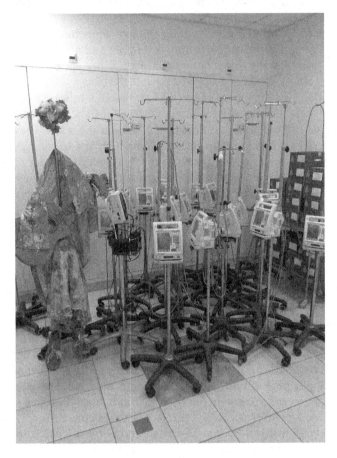

Figure 1.1 The scarecrow, "Sheba" hospital oncology, 2021.

References

Attardo, Salvatore (1997). The semantic foundations of cognitive theories of humor. *Humor: International Journal of Humor Research*, 10(4) 395–420. doi:10.1515/humr.1997.10.4.395

Berk, Lee; Alphonso, Clarice; Thakker, Neha & Nelson, Bruce (2014). Humor similar to meditation enhances EEG power spectral density of gamma wave band activity (31–40Hz) and synchrony (684.5). *The FASEB Journal*, 28: 684.5. doi:10.1096/fasebj.28.1_supplement.684.5

Christoff, Maria & Dauphin, Barry (2017). Freud's theory of humor. In V. Zeigler-Hill, T.K. Shackelford (eds.), *Encyclopedia of Personality and*

Individual Differences, Springer International Publishing. doi:10.1007/978-3-319-28099-8_588-1

Gervais, Matthew & Wilson, David Sloan (2005). The evolution and functions of laughter and humor: A synthetic approach. *The Quarterly Review of Biology*, 80(4) 395–430. doi:10.1086/498281

Harari, Yuval Noah (2013). *A Brief History of Mankind*. Kinneret, Zmora-Bitan, Dvir; Or Yehuda, Israel.

Lippitt, John (1994). Humour and incongruity. *Cogito*, 8(2) 147–153. doi:10.5840/cogito19948227

Lippitt, John (1995a). Humour and superiority. *Cogito*, 9(1) 54–61. doi:10.5840/cogito19959146

Lippitt, John (1995b). Humour and release. *Cogito*, 9(2) 169–176. doi:10.5840/cogito19959229

Lippitt, John (1996). Humour and release. *Cogito*, 10(1) 63–72. doi:10.5840/cogito199610145

Malhotra, Meeta & Thapa, Komilla (2015). Religion and coping with caregiving stress. *International Journal of Multidisciplinary and Current Research*, vol.3. ISSN: 2321–3124 Available at: http://ijmcr.com

Raviv, Amnon (2018). *Medical Clowning: The Healing Performance*. London, New York: Seagull Books.

2 The birth of a new profession

The invitation in 1986 by Virginia Kcim (who was in charge of development at the Children's Hospital in New York) to Michael Christensen and his friends from the Big Apple Circus to perform for the hospitalized children initiated a project that would lead to the profession of medical clowning. Michael Christensen began entering children's wards with his fellow clowns in 1986, and the profession soon spread to many countries all over the world over the following years (Christensen 2020).

Before 1986, clowns and entertainers would often visit hospitals to amuse the hospitalized. In 1908, an article was published on the front page of the Parisian newspaper *Le Petit Journal* accompanied by an illustration, about clowns performing in a children's ward in London, almost 80 years before the clowns of the Big Apple Circus. One can safely assume that there were clowns performing in hospitals long before the article in the French newspaper. However, the clowns of the Big Apple Circus began to come regularly and for a fee rather than occasionally on a volunteer basis. A new profession was born called "medical clowning." Other variations of the name include "healthcare clowning," "therapeutic clowning," or "clinic clowning," and more. Within a few years, the "clown care unit" of the Big Apple Circus began visiting a large number of hospitals. The salaries of the medical clowns were paid from donations collected for this purpose. As the number of hospitals increased steadily, many clowns joined the unit to meet the needs that arose.

Some of these clowns would move to other countries in the 1990s, where they established medical clown organizations. Caroline Simonds founded a clown organization in France in 1991; Laura Fernandez in Germany; Vladimir Olshansky in Italy; and Wellington Nogueira Santos in Brazil.

During the last decade of the 20th century, three large umbrella organizations for medical clowns were founded that operated in several

DOI: 10.4324/9781003362302-2

countries. The Clinic-Clowns were active in Belgium, Holland, and Austria, and later also in Japan. Rote Nazen International (founded by Monica Culen together with Giora Seeliger) worked in Austria, Slovenia, Slovakia, Hungary, Czech Republic, Lithuania, Poland, Germany, and Croatia, and later also in Jordan and the Palestinian Authority. Theodora Children's Charity (founded by André and Jan Poulie) worked in Switzerland, Spain, Turkey, Belarus, Italy, France, and later in China. Today, alongside the large organizations, dozens of professional medical clown organizations (and those of volunteers) operate in many of the countries around the world. In Canada, the activity of the medical clowns began with Karen Ridd, Paul Hooson, and Bernie Warren; in Australia, the local clown organization founded by Peter Spitzer is now managed by Jo Cohen together with David Symons; while in New Zealand, Thomas Pretschner directs the medical clown organization.

The film *Patch Adams* (1998) starring Robin Williams, contributed greatly to broad recognition of medical clowning. The film tells the story of Hunter "Patch" Adams, physician and activist, who worked and preached about his approach of empathetic medicine, closeness and humor between doctors and patients since the 1970s. He strove to advance an egalitarian society of solidarity that is not based on money and power. Patch founded a not-for-profit hospital in West Virginia, and for decades has been traveling the world together with volunteers, performing in orphanages and hospitals, and spreading the message of empathic healing.

In 2002, Patch Adams came to Israel for a lecture held at Assaf Harofeh – Shamir hospital. His presence and appearance in Israel stimulated the local scene and accelerated the development of professional medical clowning in Israel. That same year, the Dream Doctors organization of medical clowns in Israel was founded by Yaakov Shriqui and is currently managed by Tsour Shriqui.

Dream Doctors is a leading clown organization from two aspects. The first aspect is its approach: it developed a model in which the medical clowns are an integral part of the medical team: their work does not only take place in the hospital rooms and corridors but also and especially in the treatment rooms. The clowns take part in performing various medical procedures as an integral part of the medical care team (doctors, nurses, and technicians).

This is a new model of medical clowning that was presented at the first international conference for medical clowning that took place at Kibbutz Ma'ale Ha'Hamisha in the Judean Hills in 2011. The international conference, initiated and organized by the Dream Doctors

Project, was attended by dozens of representatives of organizations of medical clowns from many countries around the world.

Dream Doctor medical clowns are involved in many procedures such as doctor's examination, infusion insertion, blood sampling, burn treatments, chemotherapy treatments, dialysis treatments, invasive tests, x-rays, catheter insertion, ultrasound, isotope testing, gastro examination, lumbar puncture, accompanying surgeries, and dozens of other procedures. Some of the procedures medical team members even prefer to conduct, some of the painful procedures only in the presence of a medical clown – especially with children – and wait for them to arrive in the treatment room before conducting the procedure.

If the vision of this model should be credited to the managers of the project, then its fantastic implementation is to the credit of the Dream Doctors themselves, who during many years of working as partners in various procedures, specialized and created a rationale and unique ways of working, which they share in various conferences and publications with researchers and clown doctors in Israel and around the world. Let me list just a few examples: Shoshi Ofir, who for years has been working at the Padeh Hospital, Poriyah, at its center for the treatment of victims of sexual violence; Hagar Hofesh who works in the children's and premature infant wards at Barzilai Medical Center; Noam Inbar, an important figure in the children's rehabilitation wards at Sheba Medical Center-Tel Hashomer Hospital; Miki Bush and Itai Nachmias, who are working with the mentally challenged hospitalized at Shaar Menashe; and, of course, many others.

The second aspect is the connection to academia and encouraging the conduct of various academic studies related to medical clowning. The Dream Doctors Project initiated, encouraged and established a special fund which already has supported dozens of studies whose results were published in professional literature, in leading respected medical and paramedical journals. In this way, the Project added a great deal of knowledge on the subject of medical clowning. The knowledge contributed not only to medical clowns but also and especially to doctors, nurses, and the medical establishment. These studies are a necessary condition for establishing the profession of medical clowning as a legitimate and proven profession, accepted by the community and the medical establishment in the world.

The University of Haifa, Department of Theater, in an interdisciplinary program with the Department of Nursing and in collaboration with the Dream Doctors Project, opened the first track for a degree in medical clowning. Prof. Atay Citron, head of the theatre department, formulated the unique academic program that includes theoretical and practical lessons in the fields of theater, clowning, and nursing. About 20 clowns from the Dream Doctors (and other students) began their studies in 2006 in the first ever BA degree program in medical clowning. I had the privilege of teaching in this program and in other academic programs that were among the first to include medical clowning studies in their curriculum.

In 2011, I was approached by Dr. Assi Cicurel to teach medical students at the Ben Gurion University School of Medicine, Beer Sheva. Co-instructor with Dr. Yoel Tawil, the course title was "Theatrical skills and medical clowning," and was important for exposing the medical students to the field of medical clowning and how (as future doctors) they could cooperate in the best way with the clown doctors. In addition, the course provided the medical students with interpersonal communication tools through humor and empathy. I was also invited by Prof. Susanna Pendzik to teach medical clowning in the Master's Degree program in Drama Therapy at Tel Hai College in northern Israel. Prof. Pendzik and I wrote an article comparing medical clowning to drama therapy (Pendzik & Raviv 2011) which was among the first articles to examine the work of the medical clown from the perspective of an art therapist.

The presentations at the first conference inspired medical clowns around the world to collaborate with academic institutions and create new programs for the study of medical clowning, and thereby lead to the academicization of the profession. The late Helen Donnelly from Canada initiated a certificate program at George Brown College, Toronto, in 2018. Zach Steele leads a program for medical clowning at the University of Southern California. Jack Gomberg, a student from Chicago, came to Israel on a Fulbright Scholarship, to conduct a year-long study at the Rabin Medical Center, under my guidance, in collaboration with Prof. Eyal Fenig and Dr. Noam Meiri with the academic cooperation of Tel Hai College. The results of the study were published (Gomberg et al. 2020).

Many medical clown organizations have made great contributions to the profession of medical clowning, meeting with patients and their families, working with the medical staff, and conducting scientific studies on the contribution of medical clowning to the patients and the medical staff. The International Conference of Dream Doctors in 2011 launched a tradition of international conferences. Over the last ten years, similar conferences were held in Florence (2014), Lisbon (2016), Vienna (2018), and The Hague (2022).

The Medical Clowning Conference in The Hague was held in April 2022 for three days, with an average of 320 participants each day.

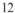

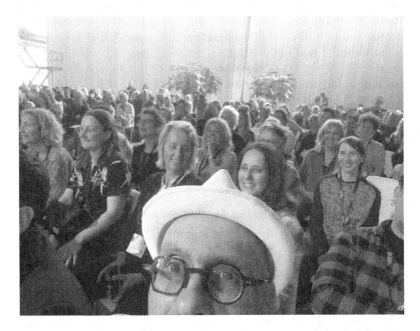

Figure 2.1 The International Healthcare Clowns' conference, held in The Hague. April 2022.

Attendees from 35 countries around the world represented many of the medical clown organizations. Dozens of medical clowns and researchers took part in workshops and lectures. The main topic of this conference (postponed several times during the year due to Covid-19 pandemic) was, of course, medical clowning during the pandemic. That is exactly what I am going to discuss in the next chapter (Figure 2.1).

References

Christensen, Michael (2020). Humanizing healthcare through humor: Or how medical clowning came to be. *The Drama Review*, 64(3) (247) 52–66.

Gomberg, Jack; Raviv, Amnon; Fenig, Eyal & Meiri, Noam (2020). Saving costs for hospitals through medical clowning: A study of hospital staff perspectives on the impact of the medical clown. *Clinical Medicine Insights: Pediatrics* 14. doi:10.1177/1179556520909376

Pendzik, Susana & Raviv, Amnon (2011). Therapeutic clowning and drama therapy: A family resemblance. *The Arts in Psychotherapy*, 38 267–275. doi:10.1016/j.aip.2011.08.005

3   Medical clowning during Covid

During the entire period of the pandemic, I worked as usual and continuously in person as a medical clown (as part of the Dream Doctors Project). In this chapter, I describe my work during the Covid-19 pandemic, 2020–2022. I analyze the impact of the pandemic on medical clowning and the effect of medical clowning on patients during this period. I began writing this book while in quarantine at home, recovering from the Coronavirus (unfortunately for me, maybe the first medical clown to have contracted the disease from patients in October 2020, even before the vaccinations were made available). In the respite imposed on me due to the illness, I had time to reflect and analyze my work as a medical clown in the various wards of the hospitals since the outbreak of Covid-19. After a stay in isolation and recovery, I returned to work in the hospital.

A threat is approaching

I will analyze the medical clowning during the pandemic according to: the timeline, the waves of the pandemic, and the different hospital wards.

Aside from my routine work in the Oncology Department at Sheba Medical Center and the geriatric wards at Herzfeld Hospital, in mid-December 2019 I joined a new study on medical clowning in the general emergency room. The study was conducted at the Shamir (Assaf Harofeh) Medical Center and included ten medical clowns from the Dream Doctors Project. The study goal was to examine whether the presence of the medical clowns in the hospital's ER during the evening and night hours lowers the level of violence (verbal and physical) by patients and their family members toward the medical team. The research was led by Dr. Efrat Danino, director of the Academic Campus for Nursing.

DOI: 10.4324/9781003362302-3

The outbreak of Covid-19 in December 2019 in the city of Wuhan, China, at first had no effect on conduct in the general emergency room at the Shamir (Assaf Harofeh) Medical Center or on the research we carried out. In fact, during its first stage, the Coronavirus had no effect on the conduct of any other ward where I worked. In the following months starting at the end of February, there were changes that took place in the triage process. From mid-March 2020, a certain tension was evident that began to be felt in the general emergency department, tension resulting from the arrival of the virus in Israel. The first cases of Covid-19 patients raised the feeling of threat. The medical clowns were at the forefront of dealing with the Coronavirus together with the medical teams, and were the "first responders" addressing patients' anxiety. One of my first jokes regarding the virus was when I announced (while coughing) that I had just returned from China... It had the effect of a slight panic and immediately a laugh of relief. Another typical joke (which disappeared as time passed and the virus stayed with us) was that the Coronavirus would not last long because it is "made in China." Although the joke is based on prejudice and is incorrect, at least it managed to make worried patients laugh.

My professional life as a medical clown became mixed up with my personal life. Shortly before I started working in the emergency room at Shamir, my father was hospitalized in the same emergency room. He had two heart attacks during those months. Following his hospitalization, I had to convince him to overcome his fear of the Coronavirus and come to the hospital for tests and treatments, which, in retrospect, saved his life.

The ER was the sharpest barometer of the changes that have taken place. Out of fear of catching the illness, people stopped coming to the ER. For a few weeks in March 2020, what was formerly an overcrowded emergency room full of people turned into a ghost ER, almost empty of patients. The medical clown group participating in the study formed a WhatsApp group where they shared experiences, stories, photos, videos, and concerns, constituting an authentic chronological record of what we went through in real time. On March 11, 2020, I joked about the study in the WhatsApp group and wrote: "The preliminary conclusion of the study is that the Coronavirus is even more effective than the clowns in reducing violence. In fact, it's very quiet here – people hardly come." But this silence was also very tense for us clowns who are supposed to overcome personal fear and reduce anxiety and make the patients who do come – laugh. One of the clowns wrote in the group: "It was a strange and interesting shift" (March 15,

2020). The next day, another clown wrote, "Not that I want to stress, but I'm stressing here." And another clown added on the same day, "Yesterday I experienced it as completely creepy." Within a short period of time, the ER changed its function once more, when it was divided into a Covid ER treating patients who arrive with symptoms, and a "normal" ER for all the rest.

There was great uncertainty at the beginning of the pandemic, and I experienced concerns and sometimes anxiety like other clowns. In fact, not only the medical clowns experienced anxiety, stress, and depression during Covid, but some of the medical team also shared these feelings (Silwal et al. 2020). How does fear affect the work of the clown doctor? The clown is afraid and celebrates. Situations of uncertainty and fear such as during the pandemic are raw material for absurd clowning. This strange paradox of fear and clowning brings carnival humor out of the clowns. The clown is at its best when on the edge. During an emergency, humor becomes crazier, wilder, and more surreal (Raviv 2012a, 2012b, 2018). Only a few days later, on March 17, one of the clowns concluded: "Here is another strange evening, the atmosphere is tense to the limit, most of the people are wearing masks, the medical team is stressed and worried and there is a strange silence."

The situation for the clown is unique and unusual. On top of the paradoxes built into the essence and routine of the medical clowning, additional paradoxes due to the pandemic joined the mix.

I will first analyze the built-in paradoxes in the normal routine of medical clowning. The arena of the medical clown's performance is the first paradox, as hospital wards are not the natural arena for a clown's performances. The medical clown tries to bring humor to a serious and humorless place, to bring joy to a place where tragic events take place, and bring vitality to the wards where death is present. The paradoxes and contradictions inherent in the medical clowns' performance are the essence of the work. But the paradoxes exist not only in the performance, but also exist powerfully between the persona of the medical clown and the person behind the clown. The persona of the medical clown sees the hospital ward as a playground and the patients as partners in play. In contrast, the person behind the clown sees the tragedy, the pain, the struggle, and sometimes the loss. All these inherent paradoxes, the "external" (between the clown, the scene, the patients, and the staff) and the "internal" (between the persona of the clown and the person behind the clown) are paradoxes and contradictions that always exist in the work of the medical clown. New paradoxes came to the fore during the pandemic.

The new paradoxes added to the clown performance during Covid

At the time of the lockdowns, quarantines, restrictions, and directives to wear masks, new internal and external paradoxes were added to the medical clown's work. In normal pre-Covid times (as well as during the pandemic), the purpose of the medical clown's work is to reduce the patient's anxiety. But the anxieties and concerns that arose during Covid are not exclusive to the patient but are also shared by the clown. Not only are both afraid, but the clown's anxieties stem from the patient her/himself (afraid of being infected by the patient) who physically caused the clown's urge not to get too close to the patient (especially if the clown feels that the protection she wears is not enough). In fact, the medical clown experiences a new internal paradox of its own – the clown fears the actual patient interaction.

External paradoxes are now added to the internal paradox faced by the clown. The physical distance of two meters that the clown is supposed to maintain, plus the mask, form a new barrier that the clown has to deal with in the interaction with the patient. The essence of the medical clown's interaction is the connection and relationship she/he creates with the patient, which sometimes includes dancing together and touching. The forced distance during the pandemic is contrary to the initial instinct of the clown who strives to create closeness and connections that have physical manifestations. In addition to this, the mask creates alienation in the patient's feeling toward the clown because it hides his face and expressions, and moreover, weakens and obscures his voice. The ability to communicate (especially with older patients who hear less well) is impaired. The clown has to raise her voice for the patient to hear her and, of course, the higher volume and tone of voice is less intimate and more alienating, making it difficult to establish contact.

Another technical paradox ensues: since the mask hides most of the facial expressions and muffles the voice and makes communication difficult, it requires getting close to the patient in order to enable connection, which is impossible since the clown must keep the "social distance" to prevent infection.

One of the first questions I asked myself when I started to conduct research on medical clowning more than a decade ago was, "What is the unity of opposites?" This is concept in philosophy used by Aristotle and Hegel, questioning what allows a thing to exist despite all its contradictions. Simply put, I wondered what enables the work of medical clowning even though it contains many contradictions. My conclusion was that the liminality in the appearance and salient characteristics of the medical clown as perceived by the patients. Liminality is the unity of opposites that makes the work possible (Raviv 2018). The seriously ill patient experiences uncertainty, having been taken out of one's daily routine upon falling ill. The experience of the hospitalized patient is liminal in the sense that the patient feels as if s/he is hanging between life and death, uncertain if release means return to normal life – or death.

Because of the patients' liminal experience and their perception of the clown as a liminal character (as someone who comes from the realms of fantasy and humor, and belongs, but at the same time does not belong to the ward) they connect with the clown. One of the main characteristics of the medical clown's appearance, perhaps the strongest component, is the costume that creates fantasy and humor. It is the fantasy that creates the clown's liminal figure in the eyes of the patient. The fantasy, like the humor, allows distancing from the immediate situation, and allows the patients to process the situation in which they deal with. In the Covid wards (not only, but especially) the clowns are forced to wear the gowns and gloves and all the protective gear that all the staff members wear and thus lose the visuality. The fantasy and humor that the medical clown's outfit inspires on normal days faded in the days of the Coronavirus as a result of the need to wear the protective outfit. With the standard outfit of staff, the clowns lose their "superpower" and the liminality of their character. Working in the Covid wards forced the clowns to find new ways to improve the standard outfit, and find alternative ways to create a fantasy that would draw the patient into alternative worlds.

At that point in time in March 2020, medical clowning in the Emergency Room at Shamir (Assaf Harofeh) Medical Center involved dealing with fear and finding new ways of working. As the months passed, knowledge about the virus accumulated, and the clowns learned over time to work with the new restrictions (such as mask, gown, and gloves). This was not the case in March 2020 when medical teams throughout the country complained about a lack of equipment. The issue also came up in the ER at Shamir (Assaf Harofeh). On March 17, one of the clowns complained about the difficulty in obtaining masks while and another clown requested that the hospital organize protective equipment for them.

As the uncertainty regarding the virus decreased, the fear naturally decreased. The vaccine that was made available significantly reduced the fear among patients and the medical teams. As the tension and fear (not to mention panic at the beginning of the pandemic) created by the virus decreased, the medical clown could create a better inter-action with the patients (within the limitations that remained for a long time, such as the mask). But the tension rose and fell for a long time because of the new mutations of the virus and the weakening of the vaccine's effect. It can be said that during the last two and a half years, a "routine" of waves of new variants, with the resulting stress and relief, affected the work of the medical clown, and impacted the nature of the interaction with the patients. The Coronavirus affected the dynamics within many families and caused more aggressive and emotional communication within the family (Lev-Wiesel et al. 2022) a factor that the medical clown sometimes had to deal with in the pediatrics departments.

At the end of each wave caused by a mutation, the tension dropped and there was no strict enforcement of wearing a mask (or the social distancing requirement) for the clowns and the patients. The feeling was of a return to the pre-Covid routine; then, as a result of a new mutation that erupted again, the tension rose, bringing with it all the consequences for the clown-patient interaction.

These waves had a special effect on the hospital geriatric wards and on nursing homes. It seemed to the patients that the plague would not end for them, and that they would have to spend the rest of their lives isolated and far from their family, a feeling that led to anxiety and depression in many of the patients and long-term residents (Kim & Kim 2021). The medical clowns had to deal with these difficult feelings, raise patient morale, and sometimes serve as a substitute for the family (in meeting the acute needs of many elderly patients). In the oncology wards the existing anxiety in dealing with cancer was increased because of the Coronavirus, which is much more of a threat to immunocompromised patients. The medical clowns had the task of reducing the increased anxiety of the doubly anxious patients suffering from both cancer and Covid, and had to work harder to strengthen the isolated patients' spirits.

Interactions in the geriatric ward during the pandemic

I would like to describe clown-patient interactions during the pandemic, at the Herzfeld Rehabilitation Geriatric Hospital in Gedera (central Israel) where patients who are in a high-risk group for the Covid-19 virus are hospitalized.

For elderly patients suffering from serious underlying diseases, the Coronavirus was particularly bad news. They were in the risk group that needs to be especially protected from the virus. Therefore, at some point the family members were forbidden to visit, which compounded their distress and loneliness. Some of them seemed to me to be clinically depressed. The loneliness imposed on patients in wards or nursing homes during the pandemic intensified the distress and depression they felt (Horesh et al. 2020). Every time I arrived, I had to wake them up from the depressive apathy that began to envelop them. Since I have known them for many months and some of them even years (for some this is "the last stop" and they will end their lives in the ward) a unique interaction was created with each of them.

When I arrive at the hospital parking lot, I dress up in the clown clothes in my car (as I always do, my habit of years). As far as I'm concerned, my clowning performance is like a site-specific performance. The sites include different wards, the ward lobby if there is one, the patient rooms, and the dining room (for the independent patients and the wheelchair-mobile, since the rest of the patients eat in bed).

On that day, I started in the first ward which was sadly depleted from the former number of patients. Recently, a number of patients were discovered to have been infected with the virus; the ward was quarantined. I know the patients personally and by name. I entered the lobby where A was sitting. Many of the patients hospitalized in the ward suffer from a mild memory problem to varying degrees of dementia. Over time, I discovered that the patients hospitalized there enjoy jokes about memory, so I told one. A laughed and Z (a patient sitting at a nearby table) called me over and offered me a tangerine (she always offers me food and urges me to eat something). I took the fruit, placed it on my head, and danced like a whirling dervish, keeping my balance, with the tangerine still on my head. Z looked especially amused at my skirt that goes up and around. For T, I danced and sang a song in Arabic while she belly-danced in her wheelchair. It's our regular top gag (an interaction that the patient really enjoys). I passed every patient in the lobby and continued to the rooms. In one of the rooms, I met A and D who remained alone amongst the four beds. (Two other patients from the same room were taken to the dialysis center in their beds). A was born in Iraq and D was born in Ukraine, so I performed a funny song that combines two songs – one in Iraqi Arabic and one in Russian, dancing between the two beds. A and D clapped to the rhythm and applauded me when I finished.

I went through all the rooms and interacted with every patient. R is an 80-year-old patient who seemed to me to be sinking into depression. She stopped smiling and turned inward. In the past, she would come to sit in the lobby of the ward, but since the pandemic began, she was found mostly sitting on her bed. She barely agreed to sing with me.

Usually, we sing old songs from the '60s. She chooses the songs and every time she remembers a sentence from the song, she gets excited. For her, remembering the words of the song indicates that her head is still working a little, which makes her happy.

From there I continued to another ward, and as soon as I entered the lobby, I began dancing with the nurse. In front of me was D, who was sitting by herself, her face sad. I approached her and started singing to her accompanying myself with the guitar. Little by little she started to move in a little dance in her chair, first for herself and then for everyone sitting in the ward. She rose and danced next to the chair with soft and beautiful movements and a smile in her eyes. It touched the hearts and was very moving for the patients sitting in the lobby who applauded enthusiastically at the end of the dance.

The Covid ward is the last ward I enter at the end of the working day. Before entering the nurses' station, there is a small room where the equipment is kept. According to the "List of protective clothing" indicated on a large plaque on the wall, I take off the normal mask and put on a special mask and another transparent mask, surgical socks on the shoes, gloves, a piece of clothing that covers the neck and head and a gown that covers the clothes.

When I'm ready, I enter the nurses' station, which is isolated from the ward by sealed windows. I press the keypad at the nurses' station to enter the ward through two doors, (sometimes together with my dear friend and clown-partner Moshe Twito). As I enter, I mime swimming, making broad arm movements in front of the sealed windows of the nurses' station and they laugh (the station with the sealed windows looks like an aquarium to me). In several rooms, severely infected Covid patients are lying in bed, unconscious and connected to an oxygen mask. Other rooms house milder patients, those who recover slowly, with whom I create amusing interactions. In the lobby of the ward there are several patients sitting on wheelchairs, who feel cured of the disease. I turn on the music and start dancing with them. As I wheel them around in the wheelchairs, I hear their laughter.

The communication is non-verbal, as it is difficult for them to hear me clearly enough through the masks and the music. The situation is amusing and one of the patients gets up from the chair and dances salsa with me (she has recovered after a long hospitalization and will soon leave the ward). I'm hot and I'm dripping with sweat under my clothes and cloak. It's hard for me to breathe with this mask after the stormy dances. I lower my energy levels in order to regulate my breathing. When I finish going through the rooms in the ward, I go out through one door (which opens by typing in a code) to a decontamination room, where I take off my robe and the rest of my clothing, change a mask, wash my hands with disinfectants and water, and exit through another door.

I feel how important it is to reach out to the isolated patients and strengthen them during this difficult time which is especially difficult for them. Loneliness is one of the main causes of distress, anxiety, and depression experienced by adults during the pandemic (Atzendorf & Gruber 2021; Santini & Koyanagi 2021). They are paying the high price of the pandemic: they are lonely, numbering among the majority of those who die during pandemic, often dying all alone in the Covid wards without family by their side.

The elderly people in the nursing homes are at the forefront of the war against the Coronavirus, and they are paying a heavy mental price because of the isolation imposed on them out of the need to preserve their lives. Keeping them safe from the virus in long isolation causes them great suffering. Closed for long months due to the closures, there are no visitors. When some of them become infected with Corona there is a closure and isolation inside their rooms. They were forbidden to go out of their rooms – even to the lobby of the department – spending long weeks without seeing their families.

At this time, once again my professional work became mixed up with my personal life. My mother was put into quarantine and isolation in the nursing home. I was afraid that she would sink into depression and so I found myself fighting for the right of family members to visit isolated parents (even if under restrictive conditions). There was no reason to prevent family visits, the parents could be seen from a distance of several meters, meetings in the open air or near the balconies. I visited my mother regularly during the quarantine. The knowledge that my mother would go into deep depression and despair if she could not see her family spurred me on to explain in every possible way why it is necessary to find ways to bring together the residents of the nursing home with their families (while keeping a distance and different solutions).

I finally came to an arrangement with the director of the nursing home: I would enter the courtyard of the nursing home, go around the building to the front of the balcony of my mother's apartment. I agreed that we would keep a distance of five meters [about 16 feet] from each other in order to maintain my mother's health. Our meetings were so important and significant for strengthening my mother's spirit – as well as my own mood – in this difficult and longtime of Covid. Medical clowning is most appreciated and deeply felt when the medical clown knows from personal experience what distress and loneliness feel like.

Online clowning

Most of the medical clown organizations in the world had to stop the face-to-face visits to hospitals by the medical clowns (at least for some period of time). Some of the medical clown organizations created alternatives to the in-person visits, using various platforms and formats such as online performances, or in-person performances from a distance, where the patients watch from across the balcony or through closed windows.

A more accurate picture of the activities of clown organizations in Europe can be obtained from the following survey: In 2020, EFHCO – the European Federation of Healthcare Clowning Organizations, in cooperation with Red Noses International – conducted a comprehensive survey of the activities of medical clowns during the Coronavirus pandemic. Out of 117 medical clown organizations that received an application to participate in the survey, 40 medical clown organizations from 21 countries of the world responded and participated in the survey. Only 36 clown organizations reported that they had to cancel or suspend the activity of medical clowns in all hospital wards. Twenty-seven clown organizations reported that their activities moved to the digital space of recorded and direct performances and interactions took place on various digital platforms. Some of the organizations physically appeared from a distance, outside the hospital building or beyond the windows (De Faveri & Roessler 2021). The activity of medical clowns online or from a great distance or through social networks is better than nothing. However, it is also clear that it is far from being as effective as in-person visits by clowns in the wards. The question being asked is why are there such policy differences in the healthcare systems in different countries referring to medical clowns' activities in hospitals during the pandemic. The differences in policy are probably rooted in the perception and recognition of the importance of the work of the medical clowns in the eyes of the policymakers. The more recognition of the importance of their work, and the higher the medical clowns' integration into an inseparable part of the interdisciplinary medical team of the hospital, the less likelihood there is that their work will be stopped during an epidemic or other catastrophe.

In an interview I conducted with Dorit Cohen, Director of Nursing at Herzfeld Geriatric Hospital, she explained why the medical clowns continued to work there as usual during the pandemic (Figures 3.1–3.7):

> Medical clowning is part of the treatment team, that is, the clowns are not seen as a group like volunteers, but as part of the overall

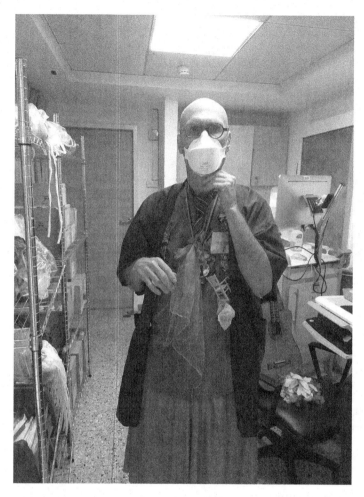

Figure 3.1 Before entering the Corona ward, the first step is replacing the mask with a special one. Herzfeld, 2021.

treatment that the patient receives from the clown (working as an integral part of the medical team). I think that the extra added value that clowns bring to patients is something that no one else from the medical team can bring. Reducing the activity of medical clowns during the Coronavirus pandemic was not even considered.

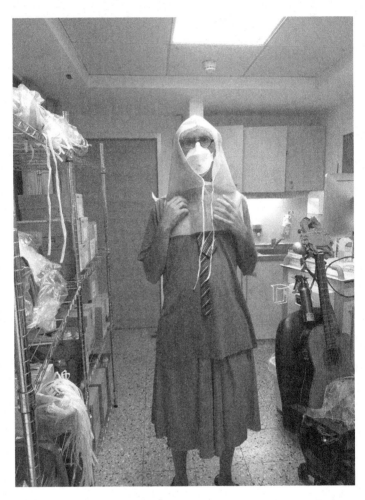

Figure 3.2 Second step before entering the corona ward is to wear a head and neck covering.

At the Medical Clowns conference held in The Hague, April 20–22, 2022 (after being twice postponed due to the pandemic), many presentations were devoted to the online work of the medical clowns during Covid-19. Since they were not allowed to enter the wards, the clowns looked for creative ways to reach patients online. By distributing iPads to patients, and through apps, the clowns were able to stay in touch with the patients online.

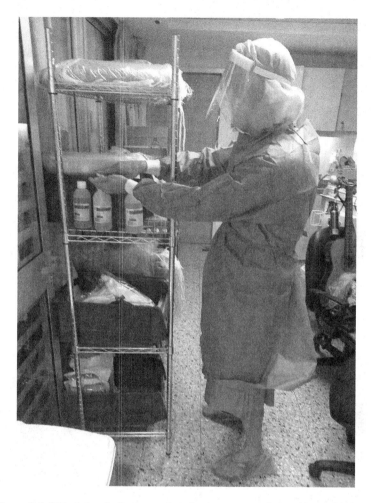

Figure 3.3 Third step before entering the corona ward wearing a cloak and shoe cover, and hand sanitizing.

The most creative way I heard about was implemented by a group from Norway led by Patrick van den Boom and Anne-Marie Cecilia Moller. With the help of a traveling robot, which consists of a column with wheels, the column topped by a screen and a camera the medical clowns could create direct interactions with patients. The clowns remained in a control room and used remote control to have the robot make its way through the wards. Using the screen and the

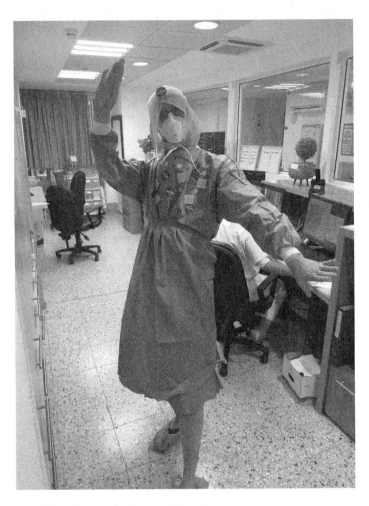

Figure 3.4 Ready to enter the corona ward.

camera by remote control, the clowns could enable both visuals and audio through the robot. In all the ways of establishing contact on-line, the clowns depended on the collaboration of the medical team (in the distribution of iPads to patients, in the accompaniment of the robot, etc.) Sometimes the collaboration was good and sometimes a little less so, or felt forced because of the many tasks the team had. For all the clowns, online work was the default and much less effective than in-person clowning in the wards. There were several clowns

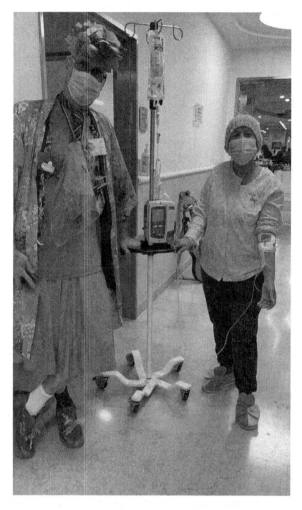

Figure 3.5 Dancing with a patient in the oncology ward at Sheba Hospital, 2021.

who noted that a small number of patients who usually experienced difficulty interacting in-person with the clowns felt more confident interacting through a screen. Most of the clowns returned to work in person (sometimes only part time) after several months and in some cases up to a year. A number of clowns did not return to regular work even two years after the outbreak of the pandemic.

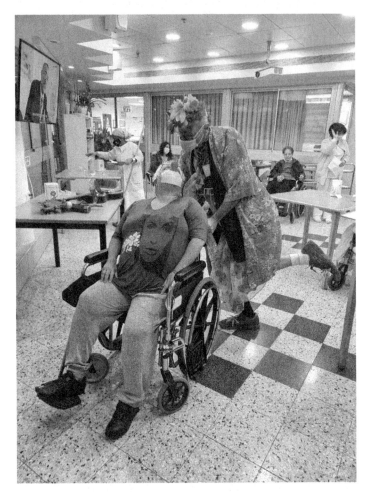

Figure 3.6 A funny interaction with a patient in a wheelchair. Herzfeld, 2020.

The study (probably the first) published on virtual medical clowning during the pandemic was by Melissa Holland (Holland et al. 2022). At the conference, Melissa presented the research carried out on the virtual interaction of medical clowns in Canada with patients diagnosed with autism, intellectual disability, voluntary muteness, borderline personality disorder, and more. Some patients responded better to online virtual clowning than to the in-person interactions of the

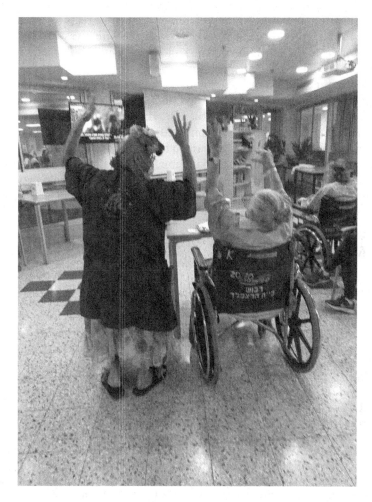

Figure 3.7 A patient dances in a wheelchair and her short clown partner. Herzfeld, 2020.

medical clowns in the ward prior to Covid. It was assumed that for some patients the encounter with the clowns through the screen was less threatening than face-to-face interactions in visits to the ward. Another study conducted in Chile showed that through online work-shops during the corona, medical clowns were able to strengthen the self-confidence of children (Valdebenito 2022). Online medical clown-ing can be an addition to the in-person medical clowning in routine times post-pandemic. For some patients with certain diagnoses, online interaction may even be preferable for various reasons. Medical clown organizations dealt creatively with the directives prohibiting visits come to the wards during the pandemic by finding different ways to keep in touch with patients online.

The main question in my opinion, the important question that medical clowns from the various clown organizations around the world should address, is how to strengthen the status of medical clowning in their country's healthcare system. Medical clowning should become an integral part of the medical team in hospitals, and continue be present on the wards even during a pandemic. It is clear that the in-person presence of the medical clowns on the ward is essential to help patients cope better with extremely high levels of anxiety, loneliness, and widespread depression.

References

Atzendorf, Josefine & Gruber, Stefan (2021). Depression and loneliness of older adults in Europe and Israel after the first wave of covid-19. European journal of ageing, 1–13. https://doi.org/10.1007/s10433-021-00640-8

De Faveri, Silvia & Roessler, Maggie (2021). Clowning during COVID-19- A survey of European Healthcare Clowning Organisations highlights the role of humour and art in the healthcare system. *Public Health*, 196 82–84.

Holland, Melissa; Fiorito, Maria-Elena; Gravel, Maï-Li; McLeod, Sarah; Polson, Jenna; Incio, Serra Natalia & Blain-Moraes, Stefanie (2022). "We are still doing some magic": Exploring the effectiveness of online therapeutic clowning. *Arts & Health*, 1–16. doi:10.1080/17533015.2022.2047745

Horesh, Danny; Kapel, Lev-Ari Rony & Hasson-Ohayon, Ilanit (2020). Risk factors for psychological distress during the COVID-19 pandemic in Israel: Loneliness, age, gender, and health status play an important role. *Health Psychology*, 25(4) 925–933. doi:10.1111/bjhp.12455

Kim, Sunhee & Kim, Seoyong (2021). Who is suffering from the "Corona Blues"? An analysis of the impacts of the COVID-19 pandemic on depression and its implications for health policy. *International Journal of Environmental Research and Public Health*, 18(23) 12273. doi:10.3390/ijerph182312273

Lev-Wiesel, Rachel; Dagan, Zehavit; Kendel, Liat; Or Amsalem, Shabtay; Lynton, Neta Rachel; From, Avital; Sokolovsky, Maayan Sapir; Weinger, Susan; Doron, Hadas & Binson, Bussakorn (2022). The impact of lockdowns during the corona pandemic on parental aggressiveness behaviors. *Journal of Loss and Trauma*, 27(5) 431–447. doi:10.1080/15325024.2021.1997207

Raviv, Amnon (2012a). Still the best medicine, even in a war zone: My work as a medical clown. *TDR: The Drama Review*, 56(2) 169–177. doi:10.1162/DRAM_a_00183

Raviv, Amnon (2012b). A clown doctor in an emergency: Theory and practice. In Avner Ziv & Arie Sover (eds.), *The Importance of Not Being Serious: Collection of Multi-Disciplinary Articles in Humor Research.* Jerusalem: Carmel, pp. 318–330 (In Hebrew).

Raviv, Amnon (2018). *Medical Clowning: The Healing Performance.* London, New York: Seagull Books.

Santini, Ziggi Ivan & Koyanagi, Ai (2021). Loneliness and its association with depressed mood, anxiety symptoms, and sleep problems in Europe during the COVID-19 pandemic. *Acta Neuropsychiatrica*, 33(3) 160–163. doi:10.1017/neu.2020.48

Silwal, Muna; Koirala, Dipti; Koirala, Sabita & Lamichhane, Anju (2020). Depression, anxiety and stress among nurses during corona lockdown in a selected teaching hospital, Kaski, Nepal. *Journal of Health and Allied Sciences*, 10(2) 82–87. doi:10.37107/jhas.210

Valdebenito, Victoria (2022). Impact of clowning with children and adolescents in confinement according to the KINDL-r Questionnaire. *Research Square.* doi:10.21203/rs.3.rs-2042838/v1

4 Medical clowning in wartime

Not even in his worst nightmares could Jan Tomasz Rogala, a Polish medical clown from Ukraine, have imagined the war in Ukraine. He would not have found it possible to grasp what he, his family, and his neighbors were going to go through. When the war began, he was not obliged to stay in Ukraine, since he and his wife and children are all Poles, and may leave. But Jan together with his family chose to stay and help the people of Ukraine in every way they could. On September 18, 2022, I conducted a video interview with him (which was interrupted by an alarm that warned of a rocket attack, according to Jan the sixth or seventh alarm for that day).

Jan and his family live in the city of Dnipro. For the past 15 years he has been working as a medical clown at the city hospital. Before the pandemic, they numbered 25 clowns, of which 21 were volunteers and four were salaried workers. During the Covid pandemic, most of the volunteers left. Except for a few months (when their work was stopped) they worked at the hospital all throughout Covid. On February 24, 2022, the day of the Russian invasion, they woke up at 5:30 a.m., terrified by the explosions in the city. Chaos ensued, and many people fled to Poland.

Jan manages the medical clowning as part of a charity that deals with helping the community in various ways. With donations received from around the world, they set up shelters and purchased buses and an ambulance to evacuate people living on the front lines of the battles. From the beginning of the war, they evacuated thousands of people to the 16 shelters in Dnipro. Even during the evacuations, he is always wearing a red nose and maintaining clownish interactions with the evacuees. In shelters they perform as medical clowns, creating funny interactions with the children and adults. The evacuation of the people from the front was accomplished at risk to their lives, sometimes under fire, while wearing a helmet and a red nose. During one of the first evacuations, they learned that a curfew had been imposed

DOI: 10.4324/9781003362302-4

on the area. They were forced to stop the vehicle and sit in it the entire freezing winter night, without being prepared for it. During the first few months of the war, the hospital of Dnipro was evacuated, and only after a while did it begin to treat the sick and wounded in the wards that were opened in the hospital basement. Jan and his fellow clowns returned to visit the hospitalized as medical clowns.

I asked Jan what is clowning for those evacuated to shelters under fire, for those hospitalized in wartime? Jan replied that clowning is hope:

> It is a break (even if for a short time) from the tension. Clowning allows the release of laughter, allows you to relax. In the darkness you see a small light, that's the hope the clown brings in war, like a little light in the dark. Hope is the power of optimism.

Jan mentioned Helen Keller, the deaf-and-blind American writer who said that optimism does not ignore reality but sees beyond reality.

Jan continued his description: "The war makes people tough and here comes the clown – looking stupid, lost, soft and vulnerable – and the people laugh. This encounter with the clown reminds them of the good and the human. Many people we evacuated from the front and passed through our shelters are today abroad. They keep in touch and write to me," says Jan. "They write to me using my clown's name, they don't know my real name."

Ostrower (2009) argued that humor was a defense mechanism that reduced Holocaust survivors' heartache and helped them cope and survive. Frankl, himself a Holocaust survivor, wrote in his book *Man's Search for Meaning* (2006) how humor strengthened the concentration camp prisoners in Auschwitz in the fight for their survival and sanity. Humor strengthens people in the most extreme, life-threatening situations. The clown is the agent of humor and fantasy, he/she is funny, and at the same time reminds people that there is humor, that there is humanity, and there is hope. The clown connects people to their own strength and humor. Laughter also provides a physical release for accumulated tension (Wooten 1996). Mooli Lahad, founder of the International Center for Stress Prevention, Kiryat Shmona, Israel, states that the appearance of the clowns in a disaster-stricken area creates an island of resilience. The clowns come to traumatized people in disaster areas and bring playfulness and laughter, helping to recreate a sense of community (Dream Doctors 2016).

Jan recalled that recently, when they arrived at the front to bring supplies to the besieged residents, there was one girl who looked at him. He distributed supplies with a red nose. The girl could not take her eyes off him. Jan made funny faces at her from afar, and for a few minutes she was captivated, smiling, forgetting her immediate reality. At the time of writing these lines the war in Ukraine continues, one clown with a red nose, together with his fellow clowns shine a small light of hope in the darkness cast by the war.

Johnny Khbeis' story is different from Jan's. In 2011, a very brutal civil war broke out in Syria. Half a million dead, and millions of displaced and refugees are the outcome of this war that lasted for years. As a humanitarian gesture, Israel treated some of the wounded. Johnny, the medical clown from the Dream Doctors Project, was sent between 2011 and 2018 to the Ziv Medical Center in Safed, to work with the wounded who experienced severe physical and mental traumas. The reason he was chosen to work with these wounded was because he is a Christian Arab and Arabic is his mother tongue. I conducted an interview with Johnny on September 14, 2022. Unlike clowns who worked in hospitals and shelters in war zones and under fire, Johnny worked in a hospital outside the war zone. The patients who arrived had very serious injuries, some had their limbs amputated. Others lost their family in the battles, and in addition to their mental and physical trauma, they were treated in Israel which for them was an enemy country. Suddenly a clown appears in the ward, named Kokuriko. He speaks their language and becomes a central character for them in the ward. Johnny became a fatherly clown to the children. They desperately needed reassurance and hugs and he responded to this need of the children. One day a three-year-old boy came to the ward and was taken to the hospital alone. He arrived without family and without anyone being able to identify him, it was not known if any of his family was alive. Kokuriko the clown took on a task, he took a photo of the boy and sent it (through the mobile phones of other wounded patients from Syria) to try to find out if anyone recognized the boy. To his joy, they located the child's mother who survived the bombing. I asked Johnny to detail what is different and special about clowning with children in the situation of the Syrian children he met. He responded by explaining that the need of the children who experienced such great physical and mental trauma is to be sheltered and loved, and he responds to that need. Kokuriko his clown persona, became paternal and sheltering, radiating love and hope.

With the older Syrian wounded, it was different. Some were tough fighters. He changed his clown's name and in order to find a way into their hearts, to gain their trust and appreciation, the way he found was through "mindreading." This is how he established a connection with them that allowed him to have a funny and clownish interaction with them, even when they had the need to talk about politics and their difficult situation. None of them would recognize him without the clown outfit, while clowning allowed him a special connection that none of the medical staff had. Even today, years after they met, some of them still write to him and keep in touch.

In his book *The Empty Space* (1968), Peter Brook described a performance by clowns in 1946 for children (in Hamburg, Germany) just after the end of World War II. The clowns sat on a cloud and ate food. He describes the image that had a hold on reality as an answer to the need for something that was really lacking at that time.

Over the many years in which I worked with children and adults admitted to the Barzilai Medical Center, Ashkelon, Israel, I encountered many suffering from anxieties and post-traumatic stress disorder (PTSD). Combat rounds between Israel and Gaza in which rockets are fired from Gaza into civilian cities in Israel began in the early 2000s. Between December 29, 2008 and January 15, 2009, I found myself on shifts lasting many long hours in the hospital's Emergency Room, which only was partially protected. Rocket barrages fell on the city. Some also fell on the hospital grounds, and some on the street where I used to live. Getting from my house to the hospital (a matter of a few minutes on normal days) turned into a long drive with several rocket attack warning alarms, causing me to stop the car and lie on the ground, shielding my head with my hands until I heard the sound of the rockets falling. I wrote in detail about my experiences as a medical clown working with anxiety victims during wartime (Raviv 2012a, 2012b, 2018).

Medical clown Hagar Hofesh is my colleague and partner at Barzilai. Several years ago, I moved to work in other hospitals but Hagar stayed there. In the 16 years she worked as a medical clown at Barzilai, tens of thousands of rockets were fired at the hospital and the city of Ashkelon in seven rounds of combat. Hagar is probably the medical clown who has worked under fire more than any other clown in the world. I interviewed her on October 2, 2022, asking her to describe several interactions she had during the war with anxiety victims and others.

The first case she described was in the unprotected orthopedic ward. She was having a funny interaction with a wounded soldier who was resting after surgery, his leg in a cast attached to a cable fixed to the ceiling. Suddenly an alarm sounded, warning of a rocket attack. Outside the room, the nurses shouted to everyone to go down to the shelter. Hagar, who was very afraid, decided that she would not leave the soldier. She pretended to wrap her hands inside his infusion tube and they both started joking that if they survived the attack, they would get married. When the attack ended, Hagar put on a nylon bridal veil and in a funny ceremony, they "married" to the laughter of patients and nurses, and even the soldier's mother who arrived (a few minutes after the attack ended) to visit her soldier son.

In another case, Hagar described an encounter with an anxiety victim in the emergency room. The new arrival in the ER was shaking all over as she waited for treatment by the medical team, who were busy working with the many other patients in the ER. There was a warning alarm for another rocket attack. Hagar hugged the anxiety victim, trying to wrap her up and make her tremors stop. The clown and the anxiety victim stood for several minutes, hugging each other. When the alarm ended, they parted with relief.

In another case, a six-year-old girl came to the emergency room. She and her uncle were traveling in a car with the aim of fleeing north, to get out of range of the rockets. Just before leaving the city, an alarm sounded. The uncle stopped the vehicle and they prostrated themselves on the ground. The rocket fell on the vehicle, the uncle was injured and was rushed to the hospital for surgery. The girl was not physically injured but was in shock and was also brought to the emergency room. In the treatment room, the medical team tried to communicate with the girl who screamed in anxiety. The doctor took everyone out of the room except the clown. Little by little the clown was able to make contact with the girl and calm her down. The clown played all kinds of games with her: they made funny glasses out of paper and jumped in all kinds of ways and shapes. The clown managed to calm the girl down and distract her from what was happening to her.

I asked Hagar what other activities she did with the hospitalized children during the war. She brought long nylon sleeves that could be inflated. These inflated sleeves looked like a very large and long balloon and they were used in the game as rockets. The children and the clown threw their nylon sleeves at each other as they warned of the rockets that were about to land on everyone. Some of the children imitated alarm sounds in their voices, but the nurses asked to stop imitating the alarms, because it scared other children. The children enjoyed the rocket game that freed them from their fears.

Besides the games, Hagar brought lollipops and distributed them to the children, because she heard that salivation reduces anxiety. She also did a massage of light blows (stronger than caresses) to calm the tremors caused by the anxiety. Together with the children, she came up with many funny songs referring to the situation they are in. Hagar applied a great deal of physical contact and gave soothing hugs to the children.

I asked Hagar in what other ways is medical clowning during war is different and she says that during war everyone needs a clown. Everyone who passes by her wants to make contact with her, hear a joke, watch her antics or magic tricks, hear a song. Everyone stops and needs a clown. Children, adults, members of the medical team, and even the hospital management requested that the medical clowns enter their rooms and meetings to relieve the tension they are harboring. Even some of the staff members who on normal days do not connect with the clowns, in times of war ask for their proximity.

I asked Hagar if a person becomes more mentally resilient over the years under a state of war. On the contrary, many residents develop PTSD anxieties that increase with each round of combat. Hagar says that the scariest part for her was always getting to the hospital with her car, a 15-minute drive from her house. During these trips (during an alarm) she would sometimes stop the vehicle and lie on the ground not far from her vehicle. Sometimes she ignored the alarm and accelerated the car's speed. These trips were always accompanied by great fear. But what happened to her in the round of fights in May 2021 had never happened to her previously. She experienced anxiety at levels she had never known. She arrived with her car at the hospital parking lot, and before she found a parking space an alarm sounded. She got out of the vehicle and has nowhere to take shelter. Above her she saw the Iron Dome defense system intercepting the rockets. She lay down on the ground and started screaming for help, she was in a panic and didn't recognize her own voice. She didn't understand who was screaming like that (didn't recognize that it was her screaming). She was in complete panic, sure that she was going to die. When it was over, she wanted to park the car (which was standing with the engine running, not yet in park). Again, an alarm sounded and again she lay on the ground screaming in panic, saying goodbye to her children in her heart. When the second rocket attack ended, she managed to get up and park the car. On the way to the hospital, when a third alarm sounded, she started running, screaming, into the hospital where she met a social worker who took her to a shelter. The social worker calmed her down for over an hour. Only after she calmed down did she continue to the children's ward to work as a medical clown. "I was struck by anxiety," Hagar told me, "I experienced terror. I have experienced what the anxiety victims I have met over the years feel." I ask her if she managed to work as a medical clown that day, and was told "Yes." About two hours after the whole incident, she had regained her mental balance, calmed down, and was able to continue her work as a medical clown. The clowning restored her strength to herself: it turns out that the medical clowning also strengthens the clown. At the end of the work day, people had to escort her to the car because the fears returned when she finished work and left the ward's protected area. The next day she was supposed to return to work at the hospital but decided to rest at home. The anxiety she experienced erupted surprisingly. Hagar the medical clown has developed PTSD over the years like many residents of the area. One never gets used to a state of war; on the contrary, the tension and anxiety increase over the years, which also affects medical clowns.

The practical side of the work

From the experience working as medical clowns with anxiety and PTSD victims, we learned that the clown's work must be quieter than on normal days (or more controlled in terms of the noise the clown produces). Sounds of loud noise such as a balloon exploding can sky-rocket anxiety levels within a split second. A booming sound can sound like the start of an alarm and will immediately cause immense anxiety to rise. More than any other sense, hearing loud sounds can return the post-traumatic sufferer to feel immense anxiety, and this can happen even years after the war.

Anxiety victims are in varying degrees of lack of connection to reality. Medical clowning can help ground them back to the reality of the "here and now." Clown's actions and questions like what's on my nose, or on my head, and asking for help in doing magic, giving roles and "responsibilities" in doing clown's tricks or magic allow the anxiety victims to connect to the here and now and "return." In acute degrees of anxiety, the disconnection from the reality of the anxiety victim is so complete that only after a sedative injection given by the doctor will the clown be able to interact with the anxiety victim.

Singing together accompanied by a guitar (or other musical instruments) with the hospitalized creates a feeling of togetherness and shared fate. The work of the medical clown through music and clowning enables personal and community empowerment. The experience that the anxiety victims are feeling includes a sense of chaos, undermining of confidence, and belief in themselves (and in the community) in the most basic ability to survive.

For the victims, the clown is a figure that restores confidence and faith (Figures 4.1–4.5). For them, the clown is a character that represents innocence, humanity, and joy, a character that can be trusted. The

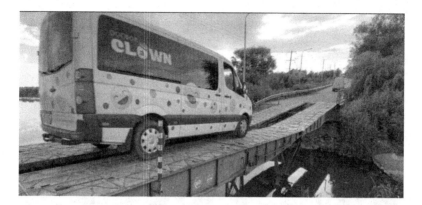

Figure 4.1 The clowns' car over a makeshift bridge. Taken in August 2022 on the way from Rohan to Kharkiv.

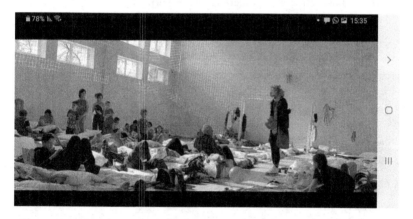

Figure 4.2 The refugee's shelter, village Voloskye. Taken in March 2022.

orthopedics ward of the Barzilai Medical Center was not protected during the wars. In the ward there were hospitalized war wounded, some also suffering from anxiety. Most of them are after surgeries and could not get out of bed. When we worked with them as medical clowns there would occasionally be an alarm of a rocket attack on the city and on the hospital. It was possible to run quickly to a protected shelter outside the ward. Since the hospitalized wounded couldn't get out of bed and run to the shelter, we would stay during the missile attack in the room with them, keep clowning around and hope for the best. We realized that

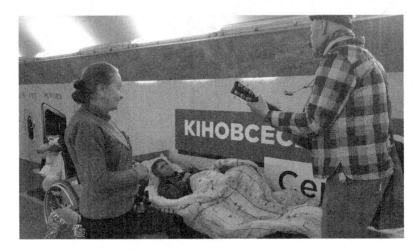

Figure 4.3 Jan in the Kharkiv metro station, April 2022.

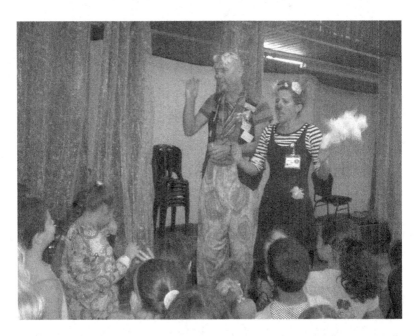

Figure 4.4 Hagar and Amnon entertaining children in a shelter, under a rocket attack, Ashkelon 2012.

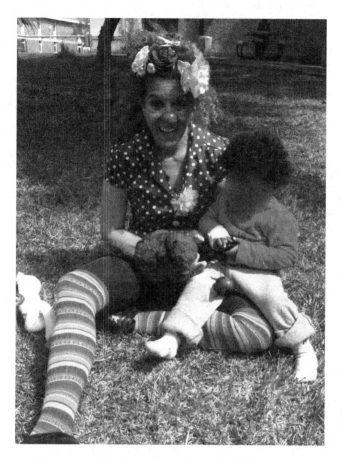

Figure 4.5 Hagar with a toddler outside the shelter during a lull in the rocket attack, Ashkelon 2012.

if we abandon them and run to take shelter, we will break their trust and we won't be able to come back to make them laugh and strengthen them as medical clowns. The fact that we stayed with them during the rocket attacks strengthened their trust and bond to their medical clowns.

References

Brook, Peter (1991). *The Empty Space*. London: Penguin.
Dream Doctors (2016). Dream Doctors, medical clowning in action: Inside the Trauma Zone. Available on YouTube, last accessed on October 15, 2022.

https://www.youtube.com/watch?v=d2Kr2kg9r9E&t=154s&ab_channel= DreamDoctors

Frankl, Viktor (2006). *Man's Search for Meaning.* New York: Beacon Press. ISBN: 0807014273

Ostrower, Chaya (2009). *Lelo humor hayinu mitabdim* [If not for humor we would have committed suicide]. Jerusalem, Israel: Yad Vashem. [Hebrew]

Raviv, Amnon. (2012a). Still the best medicine, even in a war zone: My work as a medical clown. *TDR: The Drama Review,* 56(2) 169–177. doi:10.1162/ DRAM_a_00183

Raviv, Amnon (2012b). A clown doctor in an emergency: Theory and practice. In Ziv Avner & Sover Arie (eds.), *The Importance of Not Being Serious: Collection of Multi-Disciplinary Articles in Humor Research.* Jerusalem: Carmel, pp. 318–330 (In Hebrew).

Raviv, Amnon (2018). *Medical Clowning: The Healing Performance.* London, New York: Seagull Books.

Wooten, Patty (1996). Humor: An antidote for stress. *Holistic Nursing Practice,* 10(2) 49–56. doi:10.1097/00004650-199601000-00007

5 Qualitative research on clowning in pediatrics units

In recent years, there has been a growing research interest in medical clowning. The main question that arises in these studies is in what way does medical clowning affect the patients in different medical procedures. Many studies show that medical clowning reduces patients' anxiety and pain in many and varied procedures such as botulinum toxin injection (Hansen et al. 2011); accompanying children to surgery (Golan et al. 2009); in administering anesthesia (Gomberg et al. 2020; Vagnoli et al. 2005); treating PTSD (Raviv 2012a, 2012b); treatment of sexually abused children (Tener et al. 2010); with adults suffering from dementia (Raviv 2014a); IVF treatment of women trying to conceive (Friedler et al. 2011) in adults undergoing dialysis (Nuttman-Shwartz et al. 2010; Raviv 2014c) and in the chemotherapy procedure in an oncology department (Raviv 2014b, 2018). Medical clowning has a beneficial effect on patients even beyond the procedures, that is, in the hospital rooms and in the general atmosphere of the wards (Citron 2011; Pendzik & Raviv 2011; Raviv 2013). The current study brings another layer of accumulated knowledge about medical clowning and offers new insights in the field, especially in understanding the short- and long-term patient experience after hospitalization.

The main goal of the qualitative research carried out at the Barzilai Medical Center in Ashkelon was to reach a deeper understanding of the work and roles of the medical clown in the pediatric ward.

The main methodology of the research was grounded theory construction (Charmaz 2006; Stake 2010; Strauss & Corbin 1990), a process in which the theory formed during the research is anchored first and foremost in the data that emerged from the research itself, and from that it is also supported by existing theories in the literature.

The data was collected through in-depth interviews with the medical team members in the pediatrics department through interviews with 17 doctors and 13 nurses working with the medical clowns. These

DOI: 10.4324/9781003362302-5

interviews presented a subjective perspective of the interviewees regarding the work of the medical clowns, as those who take part in the medical procedures working as a member of the interdisciplinary care team. The medical clowns have been working in the specific children's ward for over a decade. Many of the veterans among the medical team remember the ward before medical clowns worked there, and could compare the eras. The younger members of the medical team arrived at the ward when medical clowns were already working there.

The impact of the medical clowns' work

The general opinion of the doctors and nurses interviewed about medical clowning was very positive. One of the doctors expressed it this way: "I think clowning complements pediatric medicine, it's part of it, it has to be there, and I think every hospital needs at least a clown or two." One of the nurses said: "As I see it, medical clowning in my eyes works miracles and wonders." None of the staff members expressed a general negative opinion about medical clowning. When the doctors and nurses were asked to describe the impact of the medical clown's work, several themes came up.

1 The effect of the medical clown on the child.
2 The effect of the medical clown on the child's parents.
3 The clown's impact on the work of the medical team.
4 The collaboration of the medical clown and the medical team, and qualities required for good clowning.

I would now like to refer to each point in turn:

The effect of the medical clown on the child

The interviews indicated several sub-themes of influence:

1a Reducing anxiety and acute pain during medical procedures.
1b General experience of the child during hospitalization.
1c The child's experience after hospitalization in the long term.

1a Reducing anxiety and acute pain during medical procedures

The doctors and nurses pointed out the significant ability of the medical clown to distract the treated child and thus reduce

anxieties and pain. One doctor claimed: "Medical clowning makes it a lot easier for the children, it's some kind of mechanism that relieves pain."
The work of the medical clown takes place in two arenas, one is in hospital rooms and corridors, the second arena is the treatment room where the child goes through sometimes painful procedures that cause anxiety and pain (such as drawing blood, inserting an infusion, and the like). As the anxieties are greater and the pains are greater, so the ability of the medical clown to distract the child and reduce anxieties and pains has greater importance and meaning in the acute experience of the child. One doctor described his experience: "Blood tests are amazing – I have seen children stop crying...and even start smiling and laughing when the clown is present." A nurse described a girl who was very anxious about surgery and her encounter with the clown:

> There was a story about a six-seven-year-old girl who had to undergo appendicitis surgery, while the mother was an oncology patient being treated at another hospital. The girl refused to wear pajamas and objected to the wristband [hospital identification bracelet]. Every contact we had with her caused lots and lots of crying. And then the medical clown came in with balloons, and accompanied her until the moment she entered the operating room and waited for her to come out of the operating room. The girl calmed down and it was excellent, excellent.

An important issue pointed out by the team members was the medical clown's relationship with the child in the hospitalization room and escorting the child-patient to the treatment room. Creating the clown bond with the child is easier in a hospital room than in a treatment room, where the anxieties are sometimes sky high. Therefore, it is desirable that the clown makes contact with the child while still in the hospital room and accompany the child to the treatment room, so he can more easily maintain the connection and the distraction. A doctor explained it in this way:

> If a child is already lying on the table and I'm already prepping [for the procedure] and suddenly a clown comes in and starts talking to the child ... I think it has less of an effect on the child's reaction because his attention is already being tested and he doesn't pay that much attention to the clown.

However, if the clown brings the child out of the room, and starts playing with him while they're on the way, and then the staff places the child on the treatment bed while playing, it proceeds much smoother.

A nurse reinforced the point: "The child is less preoccupied with the pain and it really calms them down. They go into the treatment room with the clown more calmly." Sometimes the child is so distracted from the procedure that they do not notice that they are in the treatment room, and do not pay attention to the doctor and the prick of the needle. They are in an imaginary "other place" with the clown. A doctor described it in this way: "During a child's blood test, when the clown was playing with the boy, he didn't pay attention to me at all."

1b General experience of the child during hospitalization

Children are hospitalized for varying periods of time depending on recovery time. Their hospital experience consists of many elements such as, the illness, the meeting with the medical team, the medical procedures, the emotional consequences of the procedures, the other hospitalized children, the parents – and the medical clowns. The hospitalization experience is usually unpleasant and can cause anxiety and pain. The members of the medical team see the medical clowns as a positive factor that improves the child's experience during hospitalization in general and not only during the procedures. A doctor described his impressions of medical clowning:

> Medical clowning has consequences for the child's experience in the hospital, it's not just 'I came and suffered – that's right, I was cured, I received medicine, I feel fine – there are also positive things in a hospital. It's not just an experience of the doctor with the gown who took my blood and gave me medicine.

A nurse described the children's expectation of meeting the clowns and the way they wait for them and look for them. "The children wait for the clowns to come back later, the next day, and they look for them in the hallways and rooms." The positive experience of meeting the clown and the anticipation of their appearance keeps the child busy. The effects of the meeting with the clowns do not dissipate, but the imprint of meeting the clown remains. A doctor describes as follows:

> The children collaborate with us more due to the fact that they are with the clowns. Even if the children were with the

clowns ten minutes before we get to them, it doesn't have to be immediate. What remains is the joking game, the story they told remains in the memory.

Medical clowning creates a positive change in the child's hospitalization experience. The interaction with the medical clown has an effect on the child and has consequences for the entire hospitalization period. The effect of the clown on the child cannot be measured only by the meeting itself, but by the great impression it leaves on the child beyond the time of the meeting, throughout the length of the hospitalization, and even beyond.

1c The child's experience in the long term, post-hospitalization

Another important topic that came up in the interviews is the child's post-hospitalization experience. In what way does the encounter with the medical clown shape the experience that remains in the child's memory weeks, months, and sometimes years after hospitalization. The medical team believed that the encounter with the medical clown is greatly significant in shaping a more positive experience of the hospital stay in the child's memory. One of the nurses whose son was hospitalized (before she started working as a nurse in the ward) describes her experience as a parent of a patient:

> Three years after my 9-year-old son was hospitalized, the only thing he remembers... he does not remember being in pain and he does not remember lying with his hand raised [fixed upwards], he only remembers the clown. He keeps asking me, 'Mom, how is the clown who visited me then, the one with the green frog and the puppet he put on his fingers?' He waited all day for the clown to come.

She describes the encounter with the clown as the main experience that comes to her son's mind years after the hospitalization. Due to various medical reasons, some of the children must be re-hospitalized. The experience of the previous hospitalization is very significant for the child's level of anxiety in the child when she/he comes to be hospitalized one more time. The meeting with the medical clowns shapes the child's hospitalization experience which has a positive side: the reunion with the medical clowns. Instead of sinking into the anxieties associated with the treatment that awaits, he can remember the happy and funny meeting he had with the clowns in the previous hospitalization, and look forward impatiently to a new meeting. One of the nurses described the situation: "Many of the children are patients who return to the hospital and know the team. They remember that there are clowns and many times they ask who is the medical clown on duty today." The medical team considered the children's meeting with the medical clown to be very important, both for the sake of the general experience and the memory that the child takes with her from the hospital. One of the nurses explained: "It is important that they remember the experience of a clown in a hospital even after hospitalization."

The effect of the medical clown on the child's parents

The team noted the positive impact the medical clown has on the child's parents. The clown reduces parents' anxiety during medical procedures, especially those in which the child is in pain due to punctures for transfusion, or when blood has to be drawn and there is difficulty in finding a good vein. Any procedure that causes pain and anxiety in the child, affects the parents and causes them distress. The medical clown that draws the child's attention and reduces her anxieties and pain, indirectly reduces the parents' distress. One of the doctors described it this way: "In the procedure, the clown reduces the stress of the parents, which of course helps us." There is a reciprocal effect between the child and the parent: when the child or the parent is more relaxed, they influence each other. Sometimes the medical clown notices that the parent is very stressed and it has a negative effect on the child. In such a situation, it is worth creating an amusing clown interaction with the parent in order to reduce her anxiety, otherwise the child will not calm down either. During a procedure, calming the parent also affects the child and helps to make the procedure easier for the medical team. The ability of the medical clown to calm the parents is important, not only during medical procedures, but in general during hospitalizations and especially during the longer ones. A nurse noted: "For the parents who are frustrated that sometimes the hospitalizations are very long, the clown is not only busy keeping the child busy, they also tell jokes with the parents and it really lifts the mood." A long hospitalization in a hospital ward is not easy for the parents either. The medical team is aware of the contribution of the medical clown to raising the morale of the parents both indirectly through the children, and in the direct interaction of the clown with the parent (With, of course, antics and humor that are suitable for adults).

The effect of the medical clown on the work of the medical team

The medical team points to the great impact the medical clowns have on their work, especially during medical procedures. A nurse told me:

> The medical clowning is very helpful and succeeds in reducing children's anxiety even in all kinds of procedures we do in the ward. It distracts the child and then the doctor is freer to do the procedures of taking blood, urine tests, putting together an infusion, preparing children for surgery. It is very, very helpful.

By creating a distraction from the procedure, the medical clown succeeds in "transporting" the child to "another" place and time, thereby reducing his anxieties and distracting the child from the pain. By interacting with the child, the clown allows the medical team to be calm and focused, and to make the procedure run more smoothly. Another nurse put it this way:

> There is silence on the part of the child (who is distracted by the medical clown during the tests) it helps the nurse and the doctor, in terms of the concentration, finding the vein and the success of the procedure itself. The child is calmer, collaborates more and you hear less crying... it calms us [the team] when the child is not crying.

A doctor portrayed the impact of the presence of the medical clowns in the treatment room while performing a medical procedure on a child: "In a treatment room I am cut off from my surroundings. I always want to finish a procedure with great success and I trust the clown to calm the baby or child." Performing a medical procedure requires concentration and precision from the medical team, therefore in most cases, as the doctor described, everyone is focused on their task. The doctor and the nurse are focused on the practical performance of the procedure (for example, inserting an infusion, or drawing blood, requires concentration in order to succeed on the first attempt). The doctor stated that he trusts the clowns to calm the child. This means that the team trusts the clown to calm the child without disturbing the medical team in carrying out the procedure. In some of the procedures and in the preparation for the procedures (especially in the hospitalization rooms) there is a clownish collaboration between the medical team and the clown. The team enters the game, cooperating in the clown's antics while interacting with the child. A nurse shared her experience with me: "I'm part of the show, I collaborate with the clown to give it a broader stage." In the hospital room, a relaxed interaction with the child is possible, reducing anxiety and building trust. When the team cooperates in the clown's antics it allows better communication to take place. Such an encounter created in cooperation with the clown calms the child. The child meets the humorous side of the physician's personality as well as of the nurse who cooperate in the game. As a result, he can connect with them, feel closeness and trust them. The team indicated that the level of cooperation between them and the clown depends on their level of familiarity with the clowns and their "antics." A doctor relates: "I know where she goes, I know when she uses a certain toy, and I know what she wants with this toy, so I can enter the game together with her and the child."

Another important point pointed out by the team is the advantage of escorting the child as much as possible in moving from the hospitalization room to the treatment room. There is a great advantage in beginning the clown-child interaction in the hospital room and then continuing to interact with the child-patient in the treatment room and during the procedure. In such a case when the child is drawn into the interaction with the clown, her attention is distracted from the treatment room and the procedure. Accompanying the child increases the success rate of the clown in distracting the child and reducing her anxiety in the treatment room. A doctor phrased the results in this way: "It gives us the possibility to receive a child that is calmer, quieter, more smiling who is busy with things other than the ones we do to him."

The medical team-medical clown collaboration and qualities required for good clowning

The medical team considers the collaboration with the medical clowns to be greatly important, as well as their being an integral part of the medical team in the ward. One doctor claimed: "I think medical clowns should be here every day, they are an inseparable part of the team, and it makes it easier for us as a team at work."

Good collaboration is possible when certain conditions are met and indicated by the team members. According to the medical team, one of the main obstacles to good collaboration is the noise that sometimes accompanies the work of the medical clown. One of the nurses complained: "Too much noise, when there's a commotion in the ward and there's another noise like a clown making a loud noise, it starts to throw us off balance."

The sensitivity of the medical clown to the issue of noise is important. Clowning often naturally involves hustle and bustle, the children's enthusiasm and noise, therefore sensitivity and proper management of the issue is required from the medical clown. The medical clown has to take three factors into account regarding the noise and they are: place, time, and sensitivity of the team members. The regulation of noise (associated with the clown's work) while performing procedures in the treatment room is mandatory, since noise can distract the doctor or nurse during the procedure. Furthermore, sometimes the child screams out of fear and pain and additional noise from the clown's side can (as the nurse put it) "unbalance" the team members.

Like the general population, among the members of the medical team there are those who are more sensitive to noise, which is why it is important for the medical clown to become personally acquainted with the members of the medical team (including familiarity with the sensitivities and preferences of each one – an essential for better collaboration. As the familiarity increases and the social connection between the medical clown and the team becomes closer and closer, the team members' feeling that the clown is an integral part of the medical team in the ward increases. A nurse described the relationship:

> Our relationship [the medical team] is so good with the medical clown that I once called the medical clown when she wasn't on duty, because I had a child with extreme anxiety. The clown came especially from home. She's available, she's accessible, she's part of the team, many times it's impossible without her. Her contribution is so great in terms of doing. She is part of the team, and also in our social life beyond working hours, she is part of our WhatsApp group and joins social events.

When a close acquaintance is formed both at work and outside, the level of collaboration between the medical team and the medical clown inevitably increases and the latter becomes an integral part of the interdisciplinary and multi-professional team in the ward. When the team members were asked to describe the qualities required for a good medical clown, they described having a talent for being funny, empathetic, having an approach to children, listening ability and the ability to read the situation and react accordingly. One nurse stated:

> A medical clown needs to be able to bond successfully with the children, and also has to be able to calm us [the team] down in times of stress and distress, someone who knows how to reach out to the team as well. The clown needs to know when to take a step back, the clowns need to know their limits, when they are in close interaction with the child and when they need to take a step back and allow the team to do the work. They need to be sensitive and empathic.

Another nurse added more about empathy: "Empathy is very important here as well as a great tolerance and talent for acting, you need a lot of talent... you read the map what the child feels at that moment, and act accordingly." In addition to all these, the clown should be egoless, understand that he is not at the center of the show, but the sick child is the focus. The medical clown must be able to accept with good graces any situation in which he is required to move back in favor of the child, or meets with rejection from the child. One doctor called it flexibility: "If the clown is flexible and accepts everything with joy, even if the person in front of him does not like anything, if he is flexible, he will accept everything with an open heart."

Conclusions

The study indicates that the medical clown has the ability to generate a significant reduction in anxiety and pain, thus once again confirming a subject that has been extensively studied and resulted in similar findings (Citron 2011; Friedler et al. 2011; Gervais et al. 2006; Glasper et al. 2007; Golan et al. 2009; Grinberg et al. 2012; Hansen et al. 2011; Hendrikes 2012; Koller & Gryski 2008; Nuttman-Shwartz et al. 2010; Pendzik & Raviv 2011; Plester & Orams 2008; Spitzer 2006; Tener et al. 2010; Vagnoli et al. 2005).

This study points for the first time to a topic that has not been studied up to now: the child's memory of the hospitalization experience after hospitalization. The research shows that the medical clown has a significant positive effect on the memory of the hospitalization experience that takes shape in the child's memory after hospitalization. Children tend to have a positive memory of their hospital experience because of the encounter with the medical clowns. This has great significance among the children who have to undergo repeated hospitalizations.

The study indicates the positive impact the medical clown has on the medical team. The medical clown allows better performance of medical procedures by the team. The medical clown creates a good atmosphere for the medical team as well, relaxing and relieving the tension on the job.

The study indicates the conditions that allow good collaboration between the medical team and the medical clowns (from the point of view of the doctors and nurses). The conditions that improve collaboration are the team's familiarity with the medical clowns, their ability to connect on the one hand with the children and their companions, and, on the other hand, with the medical team. Medical clowns must have their sensitivity and ability to read the specific situation and act accordingly, and the capacity to manage the noise and chaos sometimes involved in their clowning in such a way that it does not harm the work of the medical team (Figures 5.1–5.3).

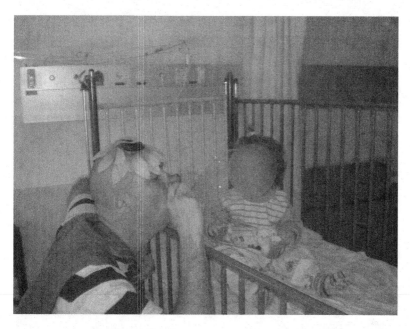

Figure 5.1 A large soap bubble distracts a cute toddler. Pediatrics Barzilai Hospital, 2007.

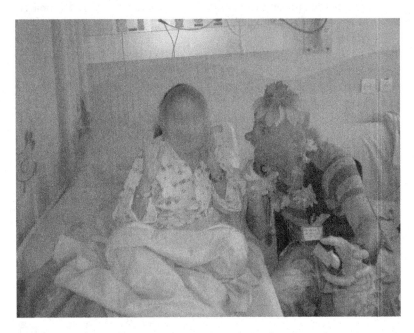

Figure 5.2 Lively interaction with a teenage girl. Sheba Hospital, 2011.

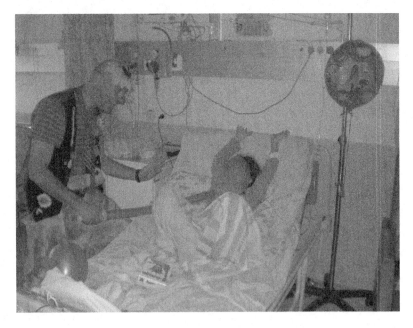

Figure 5.3 Sponge sword interaction. Barzilai Hospital, 2009.

References

Charmaz, Kathy (2006). *Constructing Grounded Theory: A Practical Guide through Qualitative Analysis.* London: Sage Publications.

Citron, Atay (2011). Medical clowning and performance theory. In James Harding and Cindy Rosenthal (eds.), *The Rise of Performance Studies: Rethinking Richard Schechner's Broad Spectrum.* London: Palgrave Macmillan, pp. 248–263.

Friedler, Shevach; Glasser, Saralee; Azani, Liat; Freedman, Laurence S.; Raziel, Arie; Strassburger, Dvora; Ron-El, Raphael & Lerner-Geva, Liat (2011). The effect of medical clowning on pregnancy rates after in vitro fertilization embryo transfer. *Fertility and Sterility* 95(6) 2127–2130. doi:10.1016/j.fertnstert.2010.12.016

Gervais, Nicole; Warren, Bernie & Twohig, Peter (2006). Nothing seems funny anymore: Studying burnout in clown doctors. In Aubrey D. Litvack (ed.), *Making Sense of: Stress, Humour and Healing.* Oxford: Inter-Disciplinary Press, pp. 77–82. Available at: https://goo.gl/cJSHmJ (last accessed on July 30, 2017).

Glasper, Edward A.; Prudhoe, Gill & Weaver, Katie (2007). Does clowning benefit children in hospital? Views of Theodora children's trust clown doctors. *Journal of Children's and Young People's Nursing* 1(1) 24–28.

Golan, G.; Tighe, P.; Dobija, N.; Perel, A. & Keidan, I. (2009). Clowns for the prevention of preoperative anxiety in children: A randomized controlled trial. *Paediatric Anaesthesia*, 19(3) 262–266. doi:10.1111/j.1460–9592.2008.02903.x.

Gomberg, Jack; Raviv, Amnon; Fenig, Eyal & Meiri, Noam (2020). Saving costs for hospitals through medical clowning: A study of hospital staff perspectives on the impact of the medical clown. *Clinical Medicine Insights: Pediatrics*, 14. doi:10.1177/1179556520909376

Grinberg, Zohar; Pendzik, Susana; Kowalsky, Ronen & Goshen, Yaron "Sancho" (2012). Drama therapy role theory as a context for understanding medical clowning. *Arts in Psychotherapy*, 1(39) 42–51. Available at: https://goo.gl/xQcHMD

Hansen, Lars K.; Kibaek, Maria; Martinussen, Torben; Kragh, Lene & Hejl, Mogens (2011). Effect of a clown's presence at botulinum toxin injections in children: A randomized prospective study. *Journal of Pain Research*, 4 297–300.

Hendrikes, Ruud (2012). Tackling indifference – Clowning, dementia, and the articulation of a sensitive body. *Medical Anthropology: CrossCultural Studies in Health and Illness* 31(6) 459–476. doi:10.1080/01459740.2012.674991

Koller, D. & Gryski, C. (2008). The life threatened child and the life enhancing clown: Towards a model of therapeutic clowning. *Evidence-Based Complementary and Alternative Medicine*, 5 17–25. doi:10.1093/ecam/nem033

Nuttman-Shwartz, Orit; Scheyer, Rachel &Tzioni, Herzl (2010). Medical clowning: Even adults deserve a dream. *Social Work in Health Care*, 49(6) 581–598. doi:10.1080/00981380903520475

Pendzik, Susana & Raviv, Amnon. (2011). Therapeutic clowning and drama therapy: A family resemblance. *The Arts in Psychotherapy*, 38 267–275. doi:10.1016/j.aip.

Plester, Barbara & Orams, Mark (2008). Send in the clowns: The role of the joker in three New Zealand IT companies. *Humor*, 21(3) 253–281. doi:10.1515/HUMOR.2008.013

Raviv, Amnon (2012a). Still the best medicine, even in a war zone: My work as a medical clown. *TDR: The Drama Review*, 56(2) 169–177. doi:10.1162/DRAM_a_00183

Raviv, Amnon (2012b). A clown doctor in an emergency: Theory and practice. In Avner Ziv & Arie Sover (eds.), *The Importance of Not Being Serious: Collection of Multi-Disciplinary Articles in Humor Research*. Jerusalem, Carmel (In Hebrew).

Raviv, Amnon (2013). Medical clowning: A training and evaluation model. *Israeli Journal for Humor Research*, 4 95–110.

Raviv, Amnon (2014a). Humor in the "Twilight Zone": My work as a medical clown with patients with dementia. *Journal of Holistic Nursing*, 32(3) 226–231. doi:10.1177/0898010113513511

Raviv, Amnon (2014b). The healing performance: The medical clown as compared to African ritual healers. *Dramatherapy*, 36(1) 18–26. doi:10.1080/02630672.2014.909865

Raviv, Amnon (2014c). The clown's carnival in the hospital: A semiotic analysis of the medical clown's performance. *Social Semiotics*, 24(5) 599–607. doi:10.1080/10350330.2014.943460

Raviv, Amnon (2018). *Medical Clowning: The Healing Performance*. London, New York: Seagull Books.

Spitzer, Peter (2006). Laughter boss. In Aubrey D. Litvack (ed.), *Making Sense of Stress, Humour and Healing*. Oxford: Inter-Disciplinary Press, pp. 83–85. Available at: https://goo.gl/dsxnux (last accessed on July 30, 2017).

Stake, Robert E. (2010). *Qualitative Research: Studying How Things Work*. New York: Guilford Press.

Strauss, Anselm & Corbin, Juliet M. (1990). *Basics of Qualitative Research: Grounded Theory Procedures and Techniques*. Sage Publications.

Tener, Dafna; Lev-Wiesel, Rachel; Lang Franco, Nessia & Ofir, Shoshi (2010). Laughing through this pain: Medical clowning during examination of sexually abused children: An innovative approach. *Journal of Child Sexual Abuse*, 19 128–140. doi:10.1080/10538711003622752

Vagnoli, Laura; Caprilli, Simona; Robiglio, Arianna & Messeri, Andrea (2005). Clown doctors as a treatment for preoperative anxiety in children: A randomized, prospective study. *Pediatrics*, 116 e563–e567. doi:10.1542/peds.2005-0466

6 Clowning around with cancer online

The impact of social media on the interaction between the medical clown and oncology patients

Over resent decades, smartphones and social media networks have transformed certain aspects of our lives and impacted the interactions of the medical clown with cancer patients in the hospital, as well. The platform proposed by social media intensifies and amplifies the encounter between the medical clown and cancer patients, facilitating integrative supportive communication with fellow patients who are "connected." Online communication contributes to shattering the stigma associated with cancer, and helps patients cope with feelings of shame and guilt that some people feel about cancer.

This chapter presents and analyzes four case studies involving the unique interactions between a medical clown and cancer patients hospitalized in the adult oncology ward and the impact of social networks on these interactions.

The internet and cancer

The internet, which burst through into our daily lives (especially since the beginning of the new millennium) facilitated a new type of communication among cancer patients. In 2003, the volume of online activities of cancer patients accessing information from ACOR – Association of Cancer Online Resources (founded by Gilles Frydman), was 115,000 hits a day (Eysenbach 2003). Over the dozen or so following years, the volume of social media activities rose significantly. Support groups on Facebook (which have become a popular means of mutual support among cancer patients) make it possible to maintain communication, transmit information, and provide mutual support (Bender et al. 2011). The online support groups for cancer patients facilitate communication in a much easier way than conducting face-to-face meetings. Online communication makes it possible to give and receive support among patients experiencing similar difficulties. The support

DOI: 10.4324/9781003362302-6

strengthens them and helps them re-focus on others' problems some of the time instead of constantly focusing on their own (Shaw et al. 2000). Monnier and his colleagues found that most cancer patients would like to communicate among themselves through the internet, and share information with their caregivers. The online communication makes personal interaction possible, including supplying information and support by caregivers (Monnier et al. 2002). Other support groups have a medical professional such as a nurse who provides support for the group (Eysenbach 2003).

Besides online support groups in social media in which cancer patients share their experiences and information, blogs also offer a platform for many cancer patients to post their monologues describing their experiences, fears and dreams. Cancer patients tend to blog to receive emotional support (and tend less to want to blog to receive information). Blogs enable significant communication by one cancer patient to others, while sharing to facilitate better emotional coping by the patients with their illness and its ramifications (Kim & Chung 2007). Patient blogs expose the general public to stories of cancer patients coping with their illness. These posts contribute greatly to shattering the stigma of cancer and cancer patients. Patients are forced to address the illness, its effects and the stigma associated with cancer which leads to shame and blame of cancer patients (Else-Quest et al. 2009; Fife & Wright 2000).

Thus, the internet and the online social media constitute an important platform for communication, information, sharing and empowerment of cancer patients. But what is the impact of the social media on the medical clown's interaction with cancer patients in hospital oncology departments? I would like to describe four case studies from my work as a medical clown in oncology departments in the Sheba Medical Center, Tel Hashomer, Israel, illustrating the impact of the internet on the patients and the interaction with the medical clown. (All names in this article are pseudonyms).

The chemo party

Dan cut an impressive figure with his height and his deep thunderous voice. About age 60, Dan had pancreatic cancer with metastases. He was receiving chemotherapy in the Oncology Day Unit, and stood out visibly with his sense of humor, optimism, and unquenchable energy. We immediately connected through a lively and loud interaction which spread joy throughout the Day Unit. Dan with his characteristically cynical humor, began his original version of a "pole dance" (with an IV pole, of course) for the patients in treatment, to the sounds of my guitar and my vocal accompaniment. His wife filmed our amusing interaction and posted photos and a video on the social media. At another one of our meetings, we decided to establish a radio-TV channel called "The Voice of Cancer," and planned how we would film our next satirical "broadcasts." The plan was for Dan to bring earphones and I would bring the microphone; he would "broadcast" and I would be the sign language "translator." We made up a jingle comprising a dance and a one-word refrain: "Caaaaaaaaaaaaancer!"

The next time we met, the skit was filmed complete with the laughter of nearby patients. When we posted it on the social media, all of the online social media friends enjoyed it. The planning and filming of these video clips became an integral part of Dan's and my interaction. At the following meetings, we posted a series of videos we called "Chemo Party 1, 2, 3" etc. with songs and dances in the Unit (during the chemotherapy treatments) with the participation of other patients. Reactions to the films showed their great popularity and sense of support among patients and others who had been exposed to the wild atmosphere of laughter in the Oncology Unit, with the film's strong vein of optimism and happy feelings

A year after Dan's tumor was found, he decided to celebrate the one-year growth of "Tumoriko" as he called it. He invited his fellow patients and healthy friends and medical staff to a party in his home. Leading the festivities with dance (mainly me) and medical grass (mainly Dan) we partied late into the night. Of course, the photos and videos from the party went up on the social media so that Dan's fellow patients who were unable to be at the party physically could enjoy it, too. The planning and filming of the videos gave Dan immense pleasure, and it was obvious he took encouragement and drew strength from the support and encouragement he received thanks to the social media.

Carnivalesque humor expresses resistance. This is low-level humor that creates a topsy-turvy world opposing the existing social order (Bakhtin 1978, 1984; Fiske 1989, 1990; Raviv 2014, 2018). The challenge of the carnivalesque laughter is not only directed at the social consensus but at the human being's existential situation. Dan's interaction with the medical clown creates carnivalesque laughter reflecting objection to what is commonly considered "acceptable behavior" in the oncology ward (quiet and orderliness as requested in the hospital can intensify the patients' feeling of alienation and other negative feelings) as well as their objection to the repression they sense following the discovery of the cancer. The expressions of carnivalesque humor in the oncology unit were intensified, receiving amplification and resonance in the virtual space of the social media networks through the stills and videos. Dan expressed his objection to his gloomy state of health by means of the funny videos. Klein has argued (Klein 1989, 1998) that all cancer patients can do in addressing the fear of death is to show that they scorn Death and resist it like a bullfighter in the arena. The carnivalesque is the emotional and physical resistance to repression.

Dan's carnivalesque expressions of resistance to his difficult situation were broadcast over the social media to other patients, resonated with their feelings and created mutual support through the comments and "conversations" generated by the videos. Dan's (and others') videos revealed the patients' humorous coping approach to illness to the healthy general public who are not hospitalized. Support, encouragement, and enthusiasm from the general public have significance for Dan and for other patients: this exposure can change the stigmatization which many cancer patients suffer from (Brown Johnson et al. 2014). Stigmas such as those associated with cancer often impact the attitude to patients, which directly impacts their emotions and capacities to cope with their illness. Some patients feel ashamed, and even guilty about having cancer. It was important to Dan to provide a very public arena to his humorous approach to coping with his illness by means of the virtual space. The humor-filled interaction of the medical clown with Dan was replicated through the social media network, disseminated through the virtual space to reach huge circles of audiences of those providing and receiving support.

A last request

I'll begin this story at the end: the final SMS I received from Rosie read,

> Dear beloved Clown-Friend, my health moves between "nightmare" and "world's greatest horror," depending on what day you ask me how I am, but at least I have the charming videos you post on the social media, and they make me feel so good inside. Keep it going, dear Clown-Friend.

A few days later, Rosie passed away. At the final stage of her illness, she remained in bed at home and did not come to the hospital, so we communicated through social media. I was aware that she was terminal, so I sent her encouraging messages, and re-posted on the social media the video her daughter filmed about a year ago. The clip shows Rosie dancing with me, stepping lightly and with great charm. We were in the Oncology ward, and other patients joined in the dance. While filming this "short," Rosie's daughter said jokingly that it's best that no National Insurance Institute official should see the film (lest they think Rosie is completely healthy and no longer needs the support money for the ill provided by the national social security institution). The daughter's comments were funny and our little dance party in the ward continued. The video is happy and hopeful. Rosie showed great flexibility and sensuousness in her dancing. When the film was posted for the first time, responses were excited and optimistic. In no way did Rosie look like someone who would lose her battle with cancer within a year. Near the end, when Rosie no longer visited the hospital, she remained "connected" with me and other patients through the social media. We posted more and more videos showing amusing and funny interactions between me and long-term patients she knew, as well as new patients. Rosie posted sharp, witty, humorous comments. In her last comment on one of the films, she said goodbye to me with a request that I continue with these videos.

A study conducted in Scandinavia showed that the internet is shaping new pathways for social communication between cancer patients – communication which shatters the feeling of isolation among cancer patients. By sharing better ways of coping with the illness, the patients are empowered (Høybye et al. 2005). While Rosie lay on a bed at home during the terminal stage of her illness, isolated from the world, she found consolation in the virtual interaction with the medical clown and other patients, some of whom she had met as they had their chemotherapy sessions together in the oncology ward. The virtual interaction made an interactive relationship possible with the medical clown and the other patients. The humorous connection distracted her from her condition. The medical clown mediated the humor and imagination for the patient not only in the hospital but also in the virtual space (through the online social media). The videos presented joie de vivre, which for Rosie presented a distraction from her pains and negative thoughts. Cancer patients often want interactions (with friends and family) which are not all about depressing subjects bringing up fears about the illness (Kvåle 2007). For Rosie, who knew that there was no hope of recovery, and was not strong enough to get out of bed, the videos were her last connection to her fellow patients in the ward. The videos depicted a joyfulness and carnivalesque humor from which she drew strength and distraction from the inevitable end.

Happy end

Hannah was a vibrant woman in her early 50s, with a great sense of humor. She recovered from her cancer after about a year of chemo and radiation treatments during which I accompanied her in the oncology unit. The tests showed no more signs of a tumor. Despite the doctors warning her not to swim in the sea during her treatment period, she refused to give up her weekly swim. Hannah impatiently awaited our meetings in the oncology ward, calling them her "light in the darkness." We had superb rapport, and our interactions were characterized by loud laughter, song, and dance. Hannah was embarrassed by her hair, which had become very thin due to the chemo, and so she covered it with a curly wig. One of her good friends always accompanied her to the treatments, and often photographed our funny interactions. The video clips and still photographs became an integral part of our encounter, and we devoted thought and planning to them. We did not have a chance to produce all of our planned videos, such as our plan for staging a "flash mob" video in the ward with the participation of other patients and medical team members. However, there was one video in which Hannah managed to get over her embarrassment about how she looked with her thinning hair, and this was the clip which was tremendously popular among her social media friends. In the short video, Hannah and I are dancing to a jazz version of "Autumn Leaves." We're dressed in matching tutus, dancing in front of other patients in the Oncology Day Unit. When the dance concluded, we made a deep bow, and Hannah took off her wig, to the laughter of the viewers. Hannah's friend filmed us, posted the video, and it received enthusiastically supportive comments.

Many cancer patients feel ashamed of being ill (McKenna Gulyn & Youssef 2010). When hair falls out due to the chemo, it is a very significant loss for patients, especially for women with breast cancer, who are coping both with the illness and with its emotional impact and effect on their self-image and feeling of femininity (Fobair et al. 2006; Schover 1994). For Hannah, the video was an opportunity to break the "shame barrier" which was part and parcel of her self-image. Sometimes, in order to liberate oneself from shame, an event with a huge number of viewers is needed (viewers in the ward and viewers from the social media networks). At the finale of the dance performance, Hannah found the adrenalin and the courage to push through the barrier.

Dancing the Can-Can

The following story also has a "happy end": "Monique" recovered from her cancer and resumed her life. A short, extremely energetic woman in her late 40s, Monique used to come to the treatments accompanied by her mother. Monique described how in our first meeting, she noticed me coming closer to her, and wondered what I was doing in the adult ward. (Medical clowns are still perceived by some patients as "belonging" to the pediatrics units exclusively), and hoped I would not come near her. But I did approach her, and we bonded very quickly. Somehow, our funny interaction generated specific characters. She took on the name "Monique" and the persona of a Can-Can dance teacher, while I was her very untalented pupil. We spoke in a French gibberish, while her mother, whom she "christened" Svetlana, filmed our dance lessons on video. Of course, the clips were posted on social media, becoming very popular among patients who watched them, since they were so amusing.

The difference between a therapist and a medical clown is that the latter is not perceived by patients as part of the medical team (Pendzik & Raviv 2011). The drama therapist "takes" the patient into the realms of the imagination while the patient is aware of undergoing a therapeutic process; in contrast, the medical clown is perceived as a clown and not as belonging to the medical team. Consequently, the patient-clown interaction is not perceived as a therapeutic process. Together with the medical clown, Monique created various personae, creating an imaginary time and place "outside" of the hospital. Our sessions became an ongoing, imaginative fictional saga. The imagination embodies natural healing powers and activates therapeutic processes (Lahad 1992). Processes of coping with crisis assisted by the imagination also occur when the patient has no awareness of the therapeutic process, and sometimes precisely because of being unaware.

The first "stage" for our "Can-Can lessons" was the ward; the second stage was the social media network for sharing the performance with many viewers, making possible interactive interaction between the medical clown and Monique and viewers. The online comments and talkbacks enabled sharing the realms of the imagination and the ridiculous aspect of the "lessons" with viewers, turning them into partners in the experience and perhaps even sharing in the therapeutic process instigated by the humor and imagination.

Media accessibility using smartphones and social networks have changed our lives over the past decade. Posting photographs and clips to the social networks at any given moment from any place by anyone presents an easy, available option. The impact upon our lives is tremendous. As a society and a community, we are linked and exposed immediately to many types of information. The social networks have changed the way in which cancer patients are able to express themselves, support, be supported, and communicate with other patients, with the medical team and the general public. The social networks have expanded the patient-medical clown interaction, expanding it through clips and photographs posted throughout the social media, facilitating communication between the medical clown and other patients, within the same hospital ward, in other units and in other hospitals. The funny videos and photos reinforce and support cancer patients by positive comments posted on the web and by the ability to maintain online interactive communication. Furthermore, these posts enable healthy people who do not enter oncology wards to be exposed to the humor and imagination of cancer patients as they face their most difficult challenges. The photos and videos on one hand allow the patients to "break the shame barrier" and lessen their feelings of self-blame associated with cancer, while on the other hand they create additional opportunities of action and events in the unique, personal medical clown-patient interaction. Often the medical clown accompanies the patient for months and even years until he recovers or passes away. Engaging in photographing stills and filming videos create additional interest and shared pleasure (brainstorming, planning what to photograph, sometimes even rehearsals) in these sessions. The social

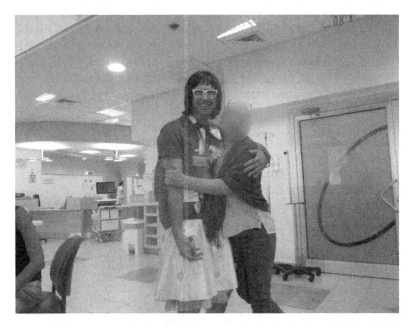

Figure 6.1 A patient who put her wig on the clown's head. Sheba Hospital, Oncology ward 2015.

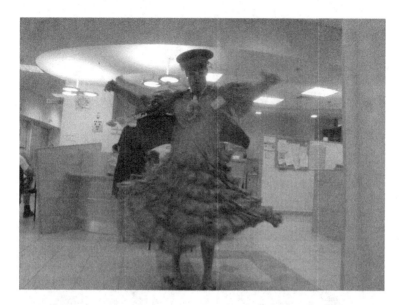

Figure 6.2 A stormy dance with a green flamenco dress. Sheba Hospital, Oncology 2017.

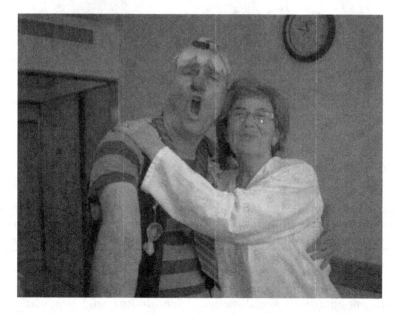

Figure 6.3 Rachel R.I.P. my family member. Soroka Hospital, Oncology 2016.

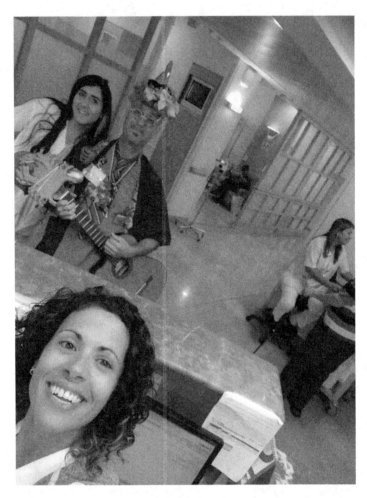

Figure 6.4 A comical encounter with two nurses. Rabin Hospital, 2016.

networks intensify and create resonance for the individual, personal interaction between the medical clown and the cancer patients, thus facilitating communication and support within a wider circle of patients and healthy people.

I would like to conclude with a humorous dialogue between the medical clown and a cancer patient which took place through private messaging on social media, demonstrating wild imagination (Figures 6.1–6.6).

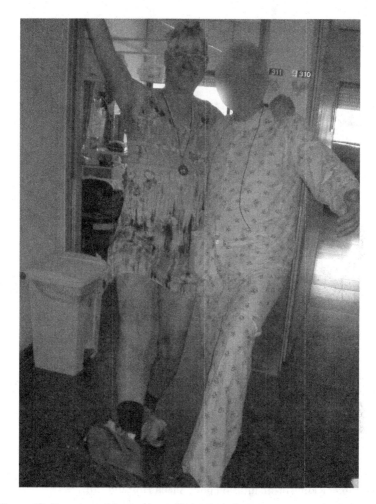

Figure 6.5 Dancing with a patient. Sheba Hospital, 2013.

MEDICAL CLOWN: When are you coming in to the department?
PATIENT: Next Tuesday, if I'm still alive by then...
MC: I'm appointing you hospital director, dead or alive...
P: I'm making you Head Nurse
MC: Maybe we should run for parliament
P: Running for parliament is running too far. Maybe we should run
    with the IV lines in the ward?
MC: So, let's also have a Unit competition on throwing IV bags ...

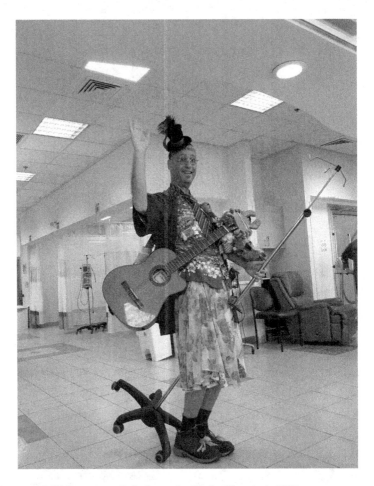

Figure 6.6 Riding on an infusion pole. Sheba Hospital, 2017.

P: … and a sniper contest using the IV needles …

MC: We'll bring a kiddie pool in here and set it up in the middle of the unit

P: … and we'll declare it a sea.

MC: We'll turn the armchairs into amphibious vehicles floating in the water … like gondolas.

P: Listen, I have a new song. It begins like this, "O Melanoma my love, O Carcinoma my sweetheart" …

MC: What a great song! We'll make a video when we meet next.

References

Bakhtin, Mikhail (1978). *Problems of Dostoevsky's Poetics* (Caryl Emerson trans.). Ann Arbor: University of Michigan Press.

Bakhtin, Mikhail (1984). *Rabelais and His World* (Helene Iswolsky trans.). Bloomington: Indiana University Press.

Bender, Jacqueline L.; Jimenez-Marroquin, Maria-Carolina & Jadad, Alejandro R. (2011). Seeking support on Facebook: A content analysis of breast cancer groups. *Journal of Medical Internet Research*, 13(1) e16. doi:10.2196/jmir.1560

Brown Johnson, Cati G.; Brodsky, Jennifer L. & Cataldo, Janine K. (2014). Lung cancer stigma, anxiety, depression, and quality of life. *Journal of Psychosocial Oncology*, 32(1) 59–73. doi:10.1080/07347332.2013.855963

Else-Quest, Nicole M.; LoConte, Noelle K.; Schiller, Joan H. & Shibley Hyde, Janet (2009). Perceived stigma, self-blame, and adjustment among lung, breast and prostate cancer patients. *Psychology & Health*, 24(8) 949–964. doi:10.1080/08870440802074664

Eysenbach, Gunther (2003). The impact of the internet on cancer outcomes. *CA: A Cancer Journal for Clinicians*, 53(6) 356–371. doi:10.3322/canjclin.53.6.356

Fife, Betsy L. & Wright, Eric R. (2000). The dimensionality of stigma: A comparison of its impact on the self of persons with HIV/AIDS and cancer. *Journal of Health and Social Behavior*, 41(1) 50–67.

Fiske, John (1989). *Understanding Popular Culture*, 2nd edn. London: Routledge.

Fiske, John (1990). *Introduction to Communication Studies*. London: Routledge.

Fobair, Pat; Stewart, Susan L.; Chang, Subo; D'onofrio, Carol; Banks, Priscilla J. & Bloom, Joan R. (2006). Body image and sexual problems in young women with breast cancer. *Psycho-Oncology*, 15(7) 579–594. doi:10.1002/pon.991

Høybye, Mette Terp; Johansen, Christoffer & Tjørnhøj-Thomsen, Tine (2005). Online interaction. Effects of storytelling in an internet breast cancer support group. *Psycho-Oncology*, 14(3) 211–220. doi:10.1002/pon.837

Kim, Sujin & Chung, Deborah S. (2007). Characteristics of cancer blog users. *Journal of the Medical Library Association*, 95(4) 445–450. doi:10.3163/1536-5050.95.4.445

Klein, Allen (1989). *The Healing Power of Humor: Techniques for Getting through Loss, Setbacks, Upsets, Disappointments, Difficulties, Trials, Tribulations, and All that Not-so-funny Stuff.* New York: Jeremy P. Tarcher/Putnam.

Klein, Allen (1998). *The Courage to Laugh*. New York: Tarcher/Putnam.

Kvåle, Kirsti (2007). Do cancer patients always want to talk about difficult emotions? A qualitative study of cancer inpatients communication needs. *European Journal of Oncology Nursing*, 11(4) 320–327. doi:10.1016/j.ejon.2007.01.002

Lahad, Mooli (1992). Story-making in assessment method for coping with stress: Six-piece story-making and BASIC Ph. In Sue Jennings (ed.), *Dramatherapy: Theory and Practice, Vol. 2*. London: Routledge, pp. 150–163.

McKenna Gulyn, Linda & Youssef, Fatma (2010). Attribution of blame for breast and lung cancers in women. *Journal of Psychosocial Oncology*, 28(3) 291–301. doi:10.1080/07347331003689052

Monnier, Jeannine; Laken, Marilyn & Carter, Cindy L. (2002). Patient and caregiver interest in internet-based cancer services. *Cancer Practice*, 10(6) 305–310. doi:10.1046/j.1523-5394.2002.106005.x

Pendzik, Susana & Raviv, Amnon. (2011). Therapeutic clowning and drama therapy: A family resemblance. *The Arts in Psychotherapy*, 38 267–275. doi:10. 1016/j.aip.2011.08.005

Raviv, Amnon (2014). The clown's carnival in the hospital: A semiotic analysis of the medical clown's performance. *Social Semiotics*, 24(5) 599–607. do i:10.1080/10350330.2014.943460

Raviv, Amnon (2018). *Medical Clowning: The Healing Performance*. London, New York: Seagull Books.

Schover, L. R. (1994). Sexuality and body image in younger women with breast cancer. *Journal of the National Cancer Institute*, (16) 177–182.

Shaw, Bret R.; McTavish, Fiona; Hawkins, Robert; Gustafson, David H. & Pingree, Suzanne (2000). Experiences of women with breast cancer: Exchanging social support over the CHESS computer network. *Journal of Health Communication*, 5(2) 135–159. doi:10.1080/108107300406866. PMID: 11010346.

7   Medical clowning and music in the wards for chronic and serious illnesses

Many studies point to music as helping to reduce anxiety and pain in patients with serious illnesses. Other studies point to humor as having a similar effect on patients. This chapter presents the medical clown as someone who successfully combines humor and music in her/his work with seriously ill patients. The chapter presents in four case studies the unique way the medical clown works with cancer patients of different degrees. From the analysis of the case studies, it appears that the medical clown's use of music helps the patients significantly in their difficult coping with the disease and its consequences.

A circus clown is a comic artist who masters several disciplines, it would not be surprising to see a circus clown who knows how to walk a tightrope, or juggle balls in the air, or play a trumpet or some stringed instrument. Sometimes the clown tries to do several things at once, in a way that seems clumsy and surprisingly succeeds (always after several unsuccessful attempts) to the cheers of the spectators. It takes a lot of skill to be able to perform various stunts in a funny way that looks clumsy and hopeless. The circus clown uses all the disciplines accepted in the circus in order to make the audience laugh. In contrast, the medical clown (according to the physical constraints in the ward, to the conventions used in the hospital, and according to the unique interaction of individual work with the patient) works differently. A large part of the disciplines of the circus clown did not enter the hospital with the medical clown. Rope walking and acrobatics, for example, were not included. In contrast, skills that are suitable for personal and intimate work with the patient and his family have been perfected. One of the important disciplines with which the medical clown works is music. Most of the medical clowns have musical instruments such as guitar, ukulele, harmonica, etc. Humor and music play an important role in empowering patients in dealing with serious illnesses and their consequences.

DOI: 10.4324/9781003362302-7

Many studies point to humor as a factor that strengthens cancer patients in their difficult dealings (Adamle & Ludwick 2005; Christie & Moore 2005; Harzold & Sparks 2006).

Other studies point to music as an important factor that helps cancer patients in their difficult coping with the disease (Ferrer 2007; Hilliard 2003; Horne-Thompson & Grocke 2008; Huang et al. 2010; Li et al. 2011; Magill 2009; O'Callaghan et al. 2007). Since these and other studies point to the ability of humor and music to help patients cope with the disease, the question arises in what unique way does the medical clown combine humor and music in order to empower the patients? I will present and analyze four case studies from my work as a medical clown in the hospital wards.

First case study: Flora

Flora (all names are pseudonyms to protect the privacy of the patients) is a 70-year-old patient in the oncology day hospital ambulatory ward, sitting on the couch connected to an IV and receiving chemotherapy treatment. Patients at the institute are often accompanied by family members or friends, especially if it is their first time at the institute for first care; Flora sat alone, collected by herself and looked fearful and sad. I approached her and indeed it turned out to me that this is the first treatment. During an amusing initial interaction in which I addressed her in gibberish steeped in a French aroma and here and there words in spoken French, it became clear to me that she does not speak French but Arabic and she was born in Iraq. Flora was still reserved and collected herself. I announced that I was going to sing her a song in Iraqi from the region of her childhood and immediately I started singing (accompanying myself with a guitar that hangs on my shoulder) a song by Verka Serduchka in Russian. Flora looked at me smiling, "Why Iraqi, does that sound Iraqi to you?" she asked amused. "Good, good sorry, here listen now" I said and started singing Mike Brant "Laisse moi t'aimer" in French of course. Flora giggled and made a dismissive motion with her hand, but joined in and sang along. Beyond the curtain in the armchair next to her, another patient joined in the singing. I asked both of them if it was okay for them to open the curtain that separates them, when I got permission, I opened the curtain and the two exchanged a few words, joking about the tutu skirt I was wearing, and continued to sing another song with me in French, this time by Edith Piaf – "Non, Je ne regrette rien." Immediately at the end of the song, I asked both of them "what they didn't like about the skirt?" and presented my white tutu skirt with two layers and pink hearts (this is a skirt that was specially sewn for me by one patient who thought I would look especially funny in a ballet skirt). My skirt is called Greta Garbo, I explained while revealing my long, hairy legs up to the thigh. Flora and her neighbor Amelia laughed out loud when I demonstrated how I danced the can-can while vigorously flapping my skirt, especially in the famous buttock movement associated with the dance. When I finished the dance and Flora calmed down from her laughter, she complained, "But you didn't sing in Iraqi." I started singing with the guitar the well-known song "Fog El Nakhil" Iraqi musicians Daoud and Saleh Al Kuwaity. Flora froze for a few seconds and looked surprised, after a moment she joined me. Her eyes sparkled as she shared with me, "This is the song I grew up listening to at my parents' house." She sang with me with great excitement. She seemed to me to be instantly traveling back in time to the realms of her childhood. When I imitated with exaggerated and ridiculous facial expressions the Iraqi singer Nazem El Ghazali (whom I once saw on YouTube) performing the song, she became very excited and explained to her neighbor Amelia that this song reminded her of her family. When I said goodbye to her, she blessed me "a thousand times" for making her happy and "bringing" her home and family.

The first thing a medical clown should do when meeting a patient is to activate his active listening, observe and understand the situation. What is the condition of the patient and what is the situation in which he is kept. The first thing that could be noticed in the described case study, is that the patient Flora is full of fear and worry, and that she is alone without the support of family or friends. An inquiry with her revealed that this was her first treatment. The initial meeting with the oncology ward, and the uncertainty about the disease, and the treatment, causes the patient great fear. A fear that is increased by the feeling of loneliness when she has no companions. Humor reduces anxiety among patients (Buxman 2008). Music also performs the same action of reducing anxiety in seriously ill patients (Thompson & Grocke 2008). When a medical clown combines humor and music when working with seriously ill patients, the effect he creates that affects and reduces anxiety is Dual. At the beginning of the interaction with Flora, the medical clown tries to "reach" her, to create a rapport between them. The medical clown strives to create a rapport with the patient because only in this way can a meaningful therapeutic relationship be formed between them. At one point the clown asked for permission to open the curtain separating Frida and her neighbor who was receiving treatment in a nearby armchair. Since Frida sat alone without companions, his goal was to connect the neighbors in order to reduce the feeling of loneliness. The medical clown has the ability to create connections between patients. It often happens that the clown connects (with various excuses) between patients who were sitting far from each other and even from different treatment rooms, because to his feelings they fit in some way and can strengthen each other during the difficult period they fell into. After a series of jokes that combine songs and jokes and after a rapport has been formed with the patient, the moment comes when the clown, at Frida's request, sings a song in Iraqi. The song touches the heart of Frida who knows it from her family home and used to sing it as a child. O'Callaghan et al. (2007) claim that there is great importance in matching the music to the patient. Familiar and close music that corresponds with the patient's identity enables processes of ventilation and a renewed affirmation of identity and the feeling of life. Frida went through a strong emotional experience through the song, an empowering experience in which she gained strength to help her deal with her situation. In fact, if we summarize the whole experience of Frida's encounter with the clown, it seems that the humor, the connection to another patient (with the help of the clown) and the music, strengthened Frida in dealing with the fears and anxieties she felt. Allow her an emotional outlet and connection to her own identity and past, and to relieve loneliness. Buxman (2008) claims that beyond alleviating loneliness, humor creates better communication and establishes good relationships, relieves stress and anger, and reduces pain. Humor and music are combined in this way, it seems only a medical clown could bring to the oncology ward.

Second case study: Daniel

I met Daniel in the small waiting room at the oncology institute, in front of the doctor's room, waiting for his turn for an examination. He was sitting on one of the chairs and his wife and daughter were sitting next to him. I contacted him and immediately recognized the heavy Spanish accent in his speech. I switched to speaking with an exaggerated Spanish accent, while playing a flamenco piece and stomping my feet to the beat. I occasionally waved the red flimsy skirt I was wearing, added hand claps to the beat and immediately went back to playing the guitar hanging around my neck. Daniel looked at me amused, he saw a medical clown, a big guy with a thin mustache in the style of the guitarist Django Rinehart, wearing a red skirt with ruffles, with a blue shirt, tie, and vest, on his head a huge colorful flower.

I told him that I lived with the gypsies in Seville in the Triana District at Tejares Street 3. I told him that I had a friend named Carmen and that I really like flamenco, both the playing and the dancing, but I have a problem with singing… I started singing in a hoarse and whiny voice as a kind of parody of flamenco singers. Daniel gave a big laugh, "Yes, yes," he said, "they really sing/cry like that." When I finished singing, he said "But I'm from Argentina". So, I started singing South American songs to him and he joined in and sang with me. His wife and daughter also joined in the singing. We sang "Guantanamera," "Besame Mucho," and "Cuando calienta el sol" Daniel sang with a smile. When we finished singing these three songs, I asked him if he knows the song "Cucurrucucu paloma." Daniel said he especially likes this song, which tells about unrequited love and how the lover's soul became a flying dove. I started playing and Daniel started singing. I felt that something special was happening, that it was a powerful moment. Daniel looked at me in my eyes and I looked in his eyes, his singing was full of emotion. I felt that the song allowed him to express an emotion that he may have been afraid to express before.

Ay, ay, ay, ay, ay cantaba,
ay, ay, ay, ay, ay gemía,
Ay, ay, ay, ay, ay cantaba,
depasión mortal moría.

Daniel sang with devotion, the song seemed to take him to another place, far from the doctor's waiting room, far from the hospital.

Fereshteh (2011) conducted a qualitative study in which he played music to patients. He found that beyond the music, the lyrics are significant for the empowerment of the cancer patient. He claims that a song with words that are relevant to the patient and create identification in him, will cause a greater therapeutic effect in the patient. One of the goals of the medical clown at the beginning of every encounter with a patient is to get to know the person standing in front of him. Familiarity with background (ethnic, geographic, family, socio-economic, education, etc.), occupation (work, hobbies, constraints, etc.), and narrative (worldview, values, dreams, etc.) or in one word that sums it up: identity. In the current case study, the medical clown recognizes the patient's Spanish accent, he first sings and plays Spanish flamenco. And then songs from South America. The rapport between the clown and the patient, built through the music and humor, involves the patient's ethnic background and language. The emerging relationship between the clown and the patient, begins with the medical clown's ability to relate to the patient's identity. Daykin et al. (2007) claim that the ability to relate to the identity of the cancer patient is a factor of great significance in the music therapy process. The therapeutic process clearly depends on the connection of the music and the lyrics (which the clown plays and sings) to the identity of the patient. Here also, as in the previous case study, the medical clown incorporates humor into the music. The appearance of the clown is funny and the demonstrations of flamenco singing and dancing were entertaining. The Spanish language is part of the patient's identity, but he stated that he is from South America. The clown and the patient sang South American songs of the patient's choice. Chuang Han Li and Young (2010) claim that patients' singing has a significant effect and causes a reduction in fatigue and an increase in relaxation and sensation. And it is possible to measure with objective parameters an improvement in the functioning of the nervous system. Ferrer (2007) claims that patients who were exposed to live music improved their quality of life, and experienced a decrease in the level of anxiety, fear, fatigue, and worry they experienced. Like music, humor also has a beneficial effect on the patient's quality of life as it reduces anxiety and pain. The beneficial effect is also on the patient's immune system through biochemical changes caused by humor and laughter and increasing the number of natural cells that fight the disease (Christie & Moore 2005). The advantage of the medical clown is that it brings both humor and music. The clown empowers the patients and their families with the help of humor and music combined with each other.

Third case study: Michelle

Michelle, a young patient about 30-years old, sat in the oncology day hospitalization department and received intravenous chemotherapy. Around her sat her sister, a close friend and a patient who was waiting for treatment. I have known Michelle for a long time from previous treatments and we had an excellent connection. I sat down next to them, since they were sitting quietly, I started to play a swing rhythm on the guitar. Michelle happily accepted and started filming everyone on video with her cellphone. Everyone started moving and improvising to the swing rhythm of the guitar. At first the improvisation consisted of funny voices made by everyone, with Michelle following with her camera the dominant improviser who took the lead. After the funny voices, her friend began improvising the words while referring to the situation, "We're not moving from here for another six minutes" (while looking at the device to see how much time is left for the treatment). Then, in the rhythm of the swing, everyone began to sing the name of the nurse (Sonia), in different melodic variations. Nurse Sonia approached with dance steps, responding to the rhythm and the song calling her name, and went to check the infusion bag hanging on a pole and attached to Michelle's arm. The treatment is not over yet, she said and danced away. The whole incident amused Michelle, who laughed out loud in response to every improvisational development of the song and the dance steps of Nurse Sonia.

Stanczyk (2011) claims that music therapy in its various options (playing, singing – active participation, and passive listening) improves the patient's condition by reducing anxiety, pain, and concerns. Michelle is a passive listener to improvisation, the words that refer to the situation in a comical way make her laugh. Actually, the song is a parody improvisation on the current situation. Unlike in Daniel's case, when the music "took" him to another place, "took" him out of the hospital, and brought him back for a few moments to his childhood and the place where he grew up. For Michelle, the music and humor presented the current situation, the current reality in a humorous way. Humor like fantasy can "take" the patient to another place, outside the time and place of the hospital and thus enable a therapeutic process. But, humor can also allow the patient to observe reality, the "here and now" from a comical perspective; thereby reducing anxiety and pain.

Fourth case study: the "Hospice Song"

After a year and a half of fighting cancer, the doctors gave up and Joe moved to a hospice for the last period of his life. He was treated with supportive palliative care in order to ease his pain. He often sat (when he felt better) together with his wife on the balcony of his small room, receiving the visits of his family and his many friends who came to say goodbye. I accompanied Joe as a medical clown during the months of his treatments and hospitalizations. We formed a strong bond. Joe had a great sense of humor that helped him deal with the difficulty and anxieties he experienced. During the months of treatment, we had a regular practice of taking videos of funny clips (sometimes songs and sometimes skits) and uploading them to social networks. Joe stuck to this habit of ours even during his stay in hospice. His wife filmed the funny video where Joe is sitting and singing, I'm next to him playing the guitar and singing with him, next to us sat his brother-in-law holding plastic crabs and shaking them to the rhythm of the song, in the style of the cheerleaders at basketball games. I uploaded the sad-comic video to the social network at Joe's request. Joe wanted to leave the world with a smile, he kept his sense of humor until his last moments. Here is the post published online, which includes the lyrics of the "Hospice Song":

> It's very pleasant here at the hospice, and the food is also quite tasty.
> Don't worry, be happy
> The neighbors are also nice, it's just a shame they disappear,
> Don't worry, be happy
> Every morning a staff member peeks, who stopped farting here,
> Don't worry, be happy
> 17 days is the average life of a hospice patient, I don't care.
> Don't worry, be happy
> I intend to live here for years, I have great conditions here
> All credit to cancer, which brought me here
> Don't worry, be happy

Five days after we recorded this song and put it on social media Joe passed away smiling and reconciled. This song was his farewell song to the world, his friends, his family, his life. He said goodbye through a humorous song that playfully winks at everyone.

Studies indicate that music also helps terminal cancer patients who are at the end of their struggle by overcoming anxiety. Music has a good and strengthening effect and improves their quality of life (Huang et al. 2010; Li et al. 2011; Magill 2009). The fourth case is a musical parody that describes the hospice experience in a comical way. The humorous song makes the situation easier not only for Joe but also for his wife and family members who are around him, and also makes it easier for those watching from a wider circle on the social network. One of the reactions to the video on the social network was from a friend: "The words have run out," to which Joe's wife replied, "When the words run out, then we laugh, sing and cry, whichever comes first."

Humor has different functions and uses for cancer patients, in the first stage humor is a mechanism to resist the disease and the situation the patient is experiencing. The humor helps the patient in dealing with the disease and its consequences. At the terminal stage when the battle with the disease is over, humor helps the patient to say goodbye to the world, his loved,ones, his family and his friends. At this stage, humor fulfills a function that helps the patient to accept and reconcile with his fate. You can call it the redemption of humor, or reconciliation and farewell with a smile. Music, together with humor, eased the parting for Joe (Figures 7.1–7.5).

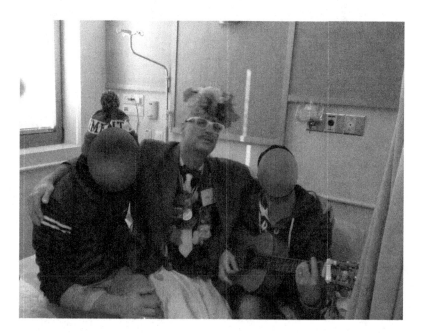

Figure 7.1 Singing in a trio. Rabin Hospital, 2015.

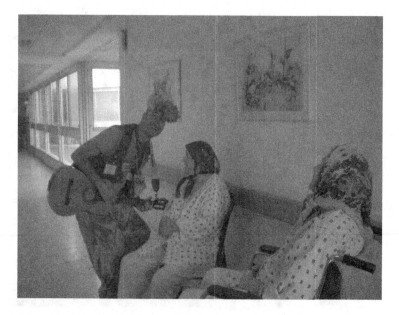

Figure 7.2 Two elderly patients with handkerchiefs. Herzfeld Hospital, 2013.

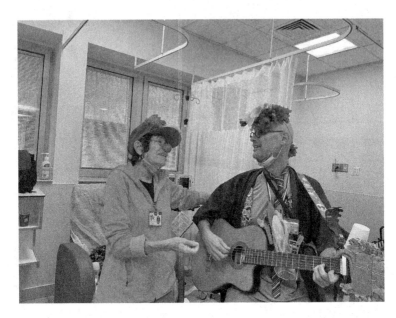

Figure 7.3 Singing with a patient who is a medical clown herself. Sheba Hospital, 2022.

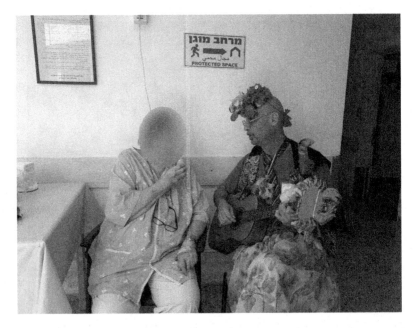

Figure 7.4 Singing to a patient who is doing an inhalation. Herzfeld Hospital, 2015.

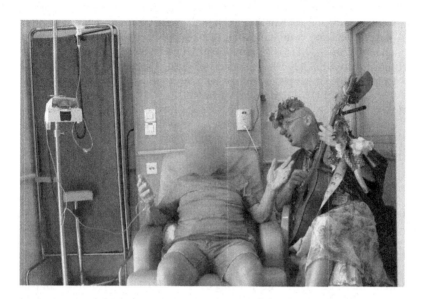

Figure 7.5 Singing with a patient in a duet. Rabin Hospital, 2015.

References

Adamle, Kathleen N. & Ludwick, Ruth (2005). Humor in hospice care: Who, where, and how much? *American Journal of Hospice and Palliative Medicine*, 22(4) 287–290. doi:10.1177/104990910502200410.

Buxman, Karyn (2008). Humor in the OR: A stitch in time? *AORN Journal*, 88(1) 67–77. doi:10.1016/j.aorn

Christie, Wanda & Moore, Carole (2005). The impact of humor on patients with cancer. *Clinical Journal of Oncology Nursing*, 9(2) 211–218. doi:10.1188/05.CJON.211–218.

Chuang, Chih-Yuan; Han, Wei-Ru; Li, Pei-Chun & Young, Shuenn-Tsong (2010). Effects of music therapy on subjective sensations and heart rate variability in treated cancer survivors: A pilot study. *Complementary Therapies in Medicine*, 18(5) 224–226. doi:10.1016/j.ctim.2010.08.003

Daykin, Norma; McClean, Stuart & Bunt, Leslie (2007). Creativity, identity and healing: Participants' accounts of music therapy in cancer care. *Health*, 11(3) 349–370. doi:10.1177/1363459307077548

Fereshteh, Ahmadi (2011). Song lyrics and the alteration of self-image. *Nordic Journal of Music Therapy*, 20(3) 225–241. doi:10.1080/08098131.2010.522718

Ferrer, Alejandra J. (2007). The effect of live music on decreasing anxiety in patients undergoing chemotherapy treatment. *Journal of Music Therapy*, 44(3) 242–255. doi:10.1093/jmt/44.3.242

Harzold, Elizabeth & Sparks, Lisa (2006). Adult child perceptions of communication and humor when the parent is diagnosed with cancer: A suggestive perspective from communication theory. *Qualitative Research Reports in Communication*, 7(1) 67–78. doi:10.1080/17459430600965924

Hilliard, Russell E. (2003). The effects of music therapy on the quality and length of life of people diagnosed with terminal cancer. *Journal of Music Therapy*, 40(2) 113–137. doi:10.1093/jmt/40.2.113.

Horne-Thompson, Anne & Grocke, Denise (2008). The effect of music therapy on anxiety in patients who are terminally ill. *Journal of Palliative Medicine*, 11(4) 582–590. doi:10.1089/jpm.2007.0193

Huang, Shih-Tzu; Good, Marion & Zauszniewski, Jaclene A. (2010). The effectiveness of music in relieving pain in cancer patients: A randomized controlled trial. *International Journal of Nursing Studies*, 47(11) 1354–1362. doi:10.1016/j.ijnurstu.2010.03.008.

Li, Xiao-Mei; Yan, Hong; Zhou, Kai-Na; Dang, Shao-Nong; Wang, Duo-Lao & Zhang, Yin-Ping (2011). Effects of music therapy on pain among female breast cancer patients after radical mastectomy: Results from a randomized controlled trial. *Breast Cancer Research and Treatment*, 128 411–419. doi:10.1007/s10549-011-1533-z

Magill, Lucanne (2009). The meaning of the music: The role of music in palliative care music therapy as perceived by bereaved caregivers of advanced cancer patients. *American Journal of Hospice and Palliative Medicine*, 26(1) 33–39. doi: 10.1177/1049909108327024

O'Callaghan, C.; Sexton, M. & Wheeler, G. (2007). Music therapy as a non-pharmacological anxiolytic for paediatric radiotherapy patients. *Australasian Radiology*, 51(2) 159–162. doi:10.1111/j.1440-1673.2007.01688.x

Stanczyk, Malgorzata Monika (2011). Music therapy in supportive cancer care. *Reports of Practical Oncology and Radiotherapy*, 16(5) 170–172. doi:10.1016/j.rpor.2011.04.005.

Thompson, Anne Horne & Grocke, Denise (2008). The effect of music therapy on anxiety in patients who are terminally ill. *Journal of Palliative Medicine*, 11(4) 582–590. doi:10.1089/jpm.2007.0193

8 Rethinking the training of medical clowns and the basics of the profession

The training of the medical clown should include the inculcation of two types of skills. The first type comprises artistic skills including improvisation, theater exercises, music, magic, movement, and juggling. The second type of skills belongs to the field of interpersonal communication and emotional intelligence. The exercises should perfect the ability to listen and observe, the ability to empathize, and the ability to establish rapport and connection with patients.

In addition, the training should include the theoretical aspects of medical clowning and familiarization with important aspects of working with patients in the hospital (prevention of infections, and more) as well as teamwork with the medical care team.

The training should include numerous observations of a large number of medical clowns at work in the hospital in different wards, with children and adults, and a long practicum that will include practical work in the hospital under the supervision of several veteran medical clowns.

It is desirable that the trainee medical clown be exposed to a considerable number of medical clowns in their work in different wards, to broaden horizons regarding the style and nature of the medical clown's work.

Medical clowning, a profession that began in children's wards, has expanded in recent decades to work in wards for adult and elderly patients. Medical clowning has become professionalized, and many medical clowns have specialized in working in specific wards and conducting specific procedures. There are medical clowns who have specialized in working with oncology patients, others in procedures for those who have been sexually assaulted, patients undergoing dialysis, chemotherapy, work in the locked wards for psychiatric patients, and many more wards.

DOI: 10.4324/9781003362302-8

The variety in ages of patients and the range of diseases with their many different procedures have changed the nature of medical clowning and require specific specializations. Therefore, the medical clown's training should be a two-stage learning process, beginning with a basic stage for all medical clowns, and a specialization stage for specific wards. Furthermore, over recent years a great deal of knowledge has been accumulated regarding the work of medical clowning during the pandemic and other extreme states of emergency, such as during war and natural disasters (tsunami, earthquake, and more).

The goal of the medical clown is to strengthen and empower the patient (encourage the connection to the life force, to humor, joy, hope, desire, love, and more). The objectives are to reduce the negative consequences caused by disease (anxiety, pain, depression, loneliness, and more). The practice of medical clowning is derived from these goals.

The way to empower and strengthen the patients is to connect with them, to find a way to bond with each and every one of them. Through a deep connection with the patients, they can be empowered. The patients should feel that they have a clown friend to whom they can feel close, that they have **rapport** with the clown, they can laugh together and fantasize a whole world that is outside the hospital ward. Patients should feel that with the clown they can celebrate life here and now despite the circumstances.

In order to reach a **rapport** with the patients, the medical clowns need the following basics in their work: The medical clown must be attentive to the patients and the situation in the ward. This is one-on-one work and each clown has to find one's unique way to reach each patient. That is why **active listening** is another basic element of medical clown work.

Authenticity, creativity, playfulness, imagination, and **humor** are other basic elements in the work of the medical clown. The clowns have to be authentic in their feelings. Acting as if you are happy (when you are not) will be a false front that will be felt by the patient (even unconsciously) and distance him/her from the clown. The skilled clown will bring all her authentic emotion into the clownish interaction. The hospital ward is a big playground for the clown, with its instruments, equipment, machines, computers, gloves, and much more. **Playfulness** and the ability to be **creative** are additional basic elements in the work. Every time the clowns use an accessory found in the ward in a context in which there is incongruity for the original function, they will create humor and fantasy.

Trust and **boundaries** are additional foundations in the work of medical clowning. First of all, there are firm boundaries in hospital work, for example, not to damage essential equipment (that's obvious!). Trust and boundaries go hand in hand. The patient is the one who sets the boundaries in the interaction with the clown. Boundaries are the line beyond which the patient will not feel comfortable, will feel hurt in one way or another, or simply will be in a situation that will not suit him/her. That is why boundaries are flexible and change according to each patient, his/her personality, and medical condition. The boundaries may change every day for the same patient because of her/his changing conditions. Boundaries include diverse areas, such as the boundaries of humor, conversation, touch, and the encounter itself. The boundaries should be sensed by the medical clown from the smallest hints given by the patient's gestures and facial expressions. The boundaries should preserve the trust created between the patient and the clown.

Trust and boundaries are also interrelated in the relationship of the medical clown and the medical team. The clown needs to gain the trust of the team. The more the team trusts the clown not to harm their work, the more the clown's freedom of action increases and the boundaries become more flexible. The team should understand that the "chaos" that the clown produces is what strengthens the patients, therefore the clown should be allowed freedom and room for action. The team has to trust the clown that the "chaos" is under control, and their work will not be affected.

What is that "chaos" that strengthens the patient? It is the **carnival spirit** that is another fundamental element in the work of the medical clown. The carnival spirit that the clown brings to the ward invites the patient to connect with the spirit of resistance to the oppression caused by the disease and its consequences. Disease depresses the body and mind, making treatment. The carnival spirit helps the patient to celebrate life here and now. It is possible to live, be happy, laugh, and dance even if you are sick, even while being treated. There is a possibility to rise up from depression and celebrate life. The carnival spirit increases the patient's mental strength and resilience. It is, not necessarily about humor or fantasy (although sometimes the carnival spirit is combined with humor and fantasy) but is about the celebration of life. For example, dancing a tempestuous dance during the treatment together with the clown is a dance that strengthens the soul.

Other foundational elements of the medical clown's work are **empathy, pleasure, sensitivity** (emotional intelligence), and what I call the **"diag-red-nosis."** The medical clown should create a shared pleasurable experience with the patient. No matter how skilled the medical clown is, if she comes to the encounter with the patient with no desire and no pleasure, the patient will feel it. If the clown is "faking it," there will be no mutual pleasure, and the encounter will not benefit the patient.

The medical clown is the only member of the medical team at the hospital whose role is to create a shared pleasurable experience with the patient. But what happens if the clown comes to the ward lacking energy and without pleasure? After all, we all have "bad days," and authenticity, as I mentioned, is an important element in the work of medical clowning. From my many years of experience, every time I arrived at the ward exhausted and lacking energy, I was re-with energy by the patients. The patients were happy to see me and their joy charged me with pleasure.

Perhaps this is the time to address the impact of the patients on the medical clown (on his/her work and especially on his/her private personal life). I can testify for myself (as well as for other medical clowns, as I learned in interviews I held with other medical clowns during which I heard similar descriptions). Working as a medical clown in the oncology wards changed me as a person. Exposure on a daily basis to the fragility of life, to suffering and death, gave me new proportions about life. This work strengthens insights and the feeling of temporality the not knowing what tomorrow will bring. Therefore, perhaps absurdly, this exposure to the fragility of life intensifies the desire to embrace life and my loved ones, the desire to use to the fullest my allotted time here on the planet. True, there is sadness in seeing patients, some of whom I connected with very much, fade away to their deaths, but with the sadness, one learns about acceptance and completion. Some of the patients inspire me enormously in the way they chose to deal with the disease and in their personality. Actually, seeing people in their times of difficulty makes me believe in the human race more than anything I see outside the hospital.

Empathy and **sensitivity** are additional fundamentals in the work. Everyone who works with patients in the hospital should be an empathic person. I heard this opinion from all the doctors and nurses I interviewed. One of the senior doctors explained the subject of empathy with a pictorial illustration: a therapist should step into the patient's shoes but not walk with them. This is a beautiful illustration that I always use when explaining empathy. The doctor's intention was that the therapist should be empathic and see the patient but not identify with him to a level that would harm his work. The same goes for the medical clown: the empathy and sensitivity the clown transmits strengthens the patient and creates a bond, but he/she must not identify with the patient and his condition in a way that would harm the clown's work and even paralyze the clown.

"Diag-red-nosis." This is a term I put together from two words – diagnosis and red nose. It refers to a basic element in the work of the medical clown, the ability to translate the data collected by active listening into correct action that will strengthen the patient. This ability rests on the clown's intelligence and emotional intelligence, on the clown's toolbox at his disposal, on his professional experience and all his knowledge and experiences as a person. I will briefly describe two cases that will illustrate my point.

I entered the hospital room where next to the bed of a young patient about ten years old I spotted a Harry Potter book. I got on a broom in the room and "rode it" as in the "quidditch" game described in the books. I immediately created contact with the girl. I translated the data (the book) and used my general knowledge about the book and my skills of improvisation to form a bond with the girl. In another case, a meeting with an elderly oncology patient who was averse to clowns presented me with a challenge of how to make contact with him. I heard from him that he is a professor of philosophy at the university and that his father, a philosopher, was part of the Viennese Circle (a group of philosophers from 1920s Vienna). I asked him if he had heard of the fireplace poker incident between the philosophers Karl Popper and Ludwig Wittgenstein. The professor looked at me in surprise and an initial connection was formed, a connection that turned into a strong clownish philosophical bond. In this case, I used my general knowledge to make the connection. Everything I know and have experienced in my life can be used by my clown self in connection with the patient. The **diag-red-nosis** is the ability to translate what is known about the patient into empowering action.

Three last fundamentals are **improvisation, gags,** and **clown interaction.** The improvisation is part of the clown interaction in which the clown mobilizes his artistic abilities to present amusing pieces created spontaneously and in real time about the current situation, or an interpretation of it, or any other topic or situation. The **gag** is anything amusing that was invented in the past and can be presented (joke, song, magic, etc.). The **clown interaction** is the patient's encounter with the clown persona (which ranges on the spectrum between a version of oneself as a clown and an invented comical character).

This is the opportunity to reflect on the issue of the persona, based on my own experiences and my observations of many medical clowns. New medical clowns have a tendency to build a comical character, a clown persona, who is very distant from the person who plays it. Over the years, the clown persona becomes closer to the person behind it, until the clown persona becomes a clownish version of oneself. And

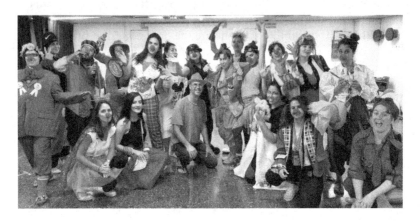

Figure 8.1 Medical clowning class. Tel Hai College, 2019.

another interesting point in this context which occurred at the beginning of my journey as a medical clown. It was clear to me that there was me, and there was my clown persona. Over the years, not only have they united, but at present it is not clear to me who is the "real me." I will explain – the clown that I am has much more freedom, he is less bound by conventions, interests and roles (father, teacher, citizen, and more). Could it be that the clown is a freer version of myself? This is an interesting question that may belong to the field of philosophy, like the question of the meaning and role of the clown in human culture since the dawn of history (Figure 8.1).

Index

Printed in the United States
by Baker & Taylor Publisher Services